AF744174

Knowledges on Thyroid Cancer

Edited by Omer Engin

Published in London, United Kingdom

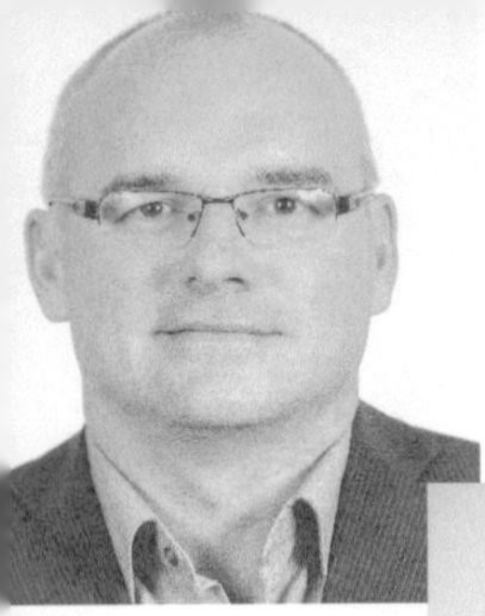
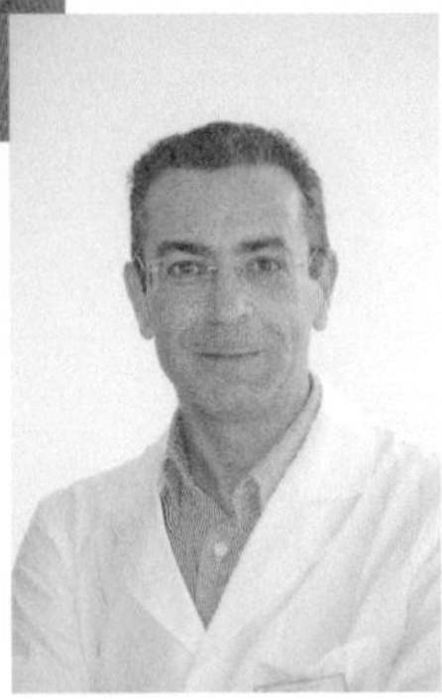
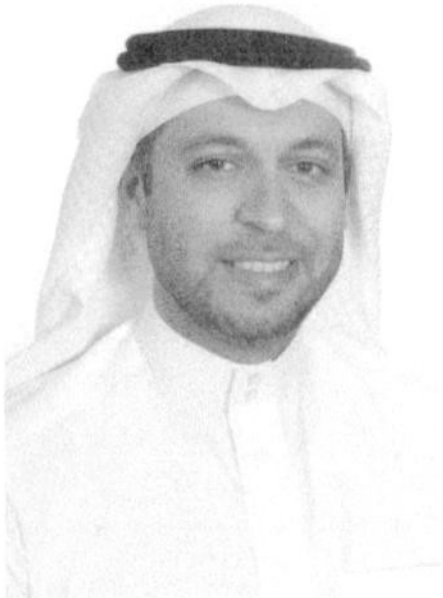
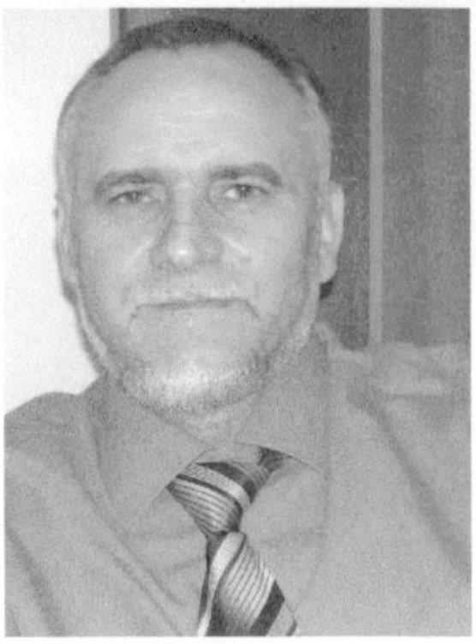
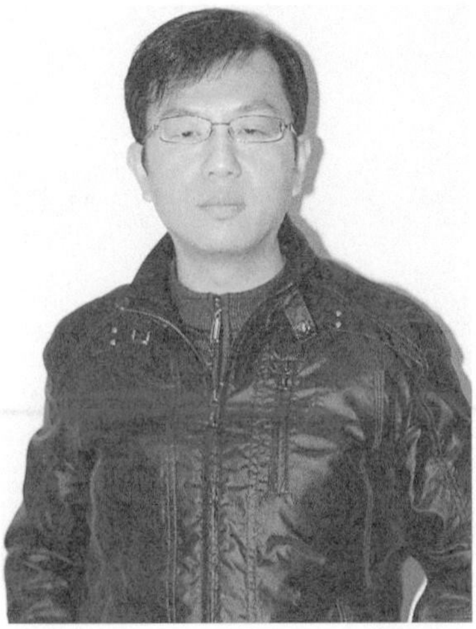
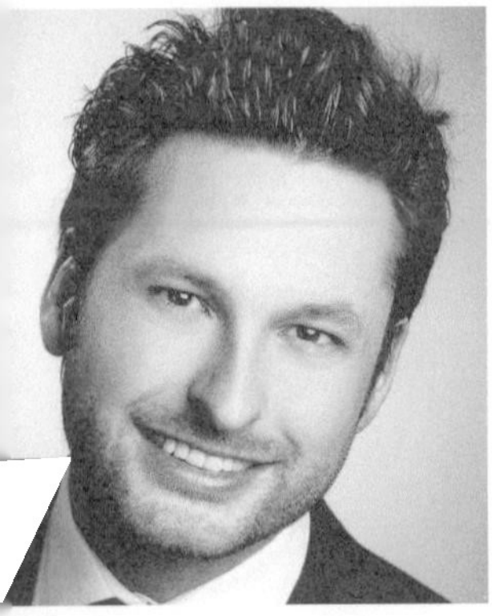
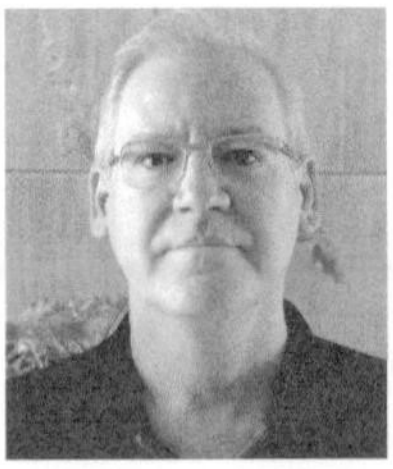

IntechOpen

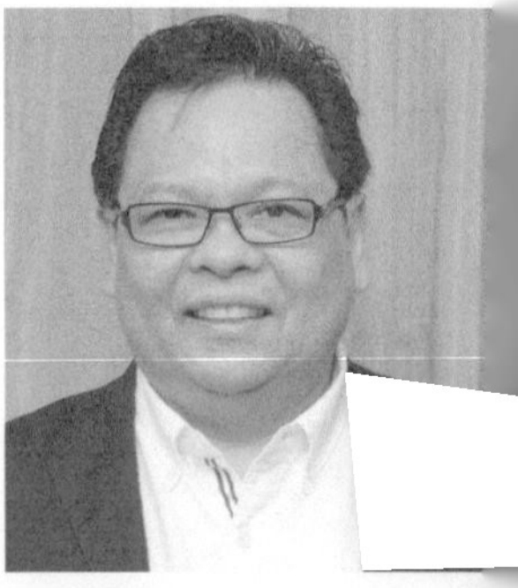
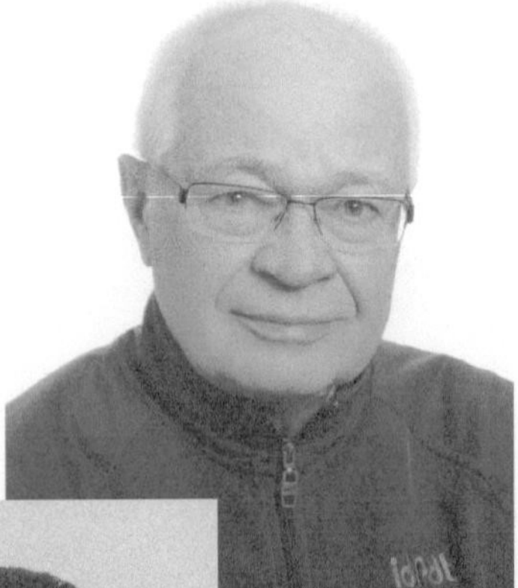
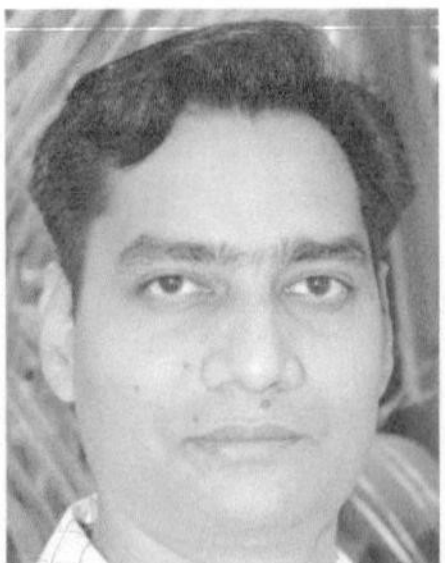
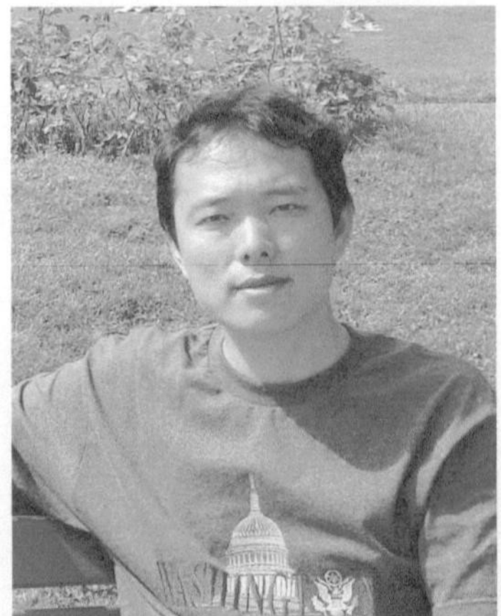
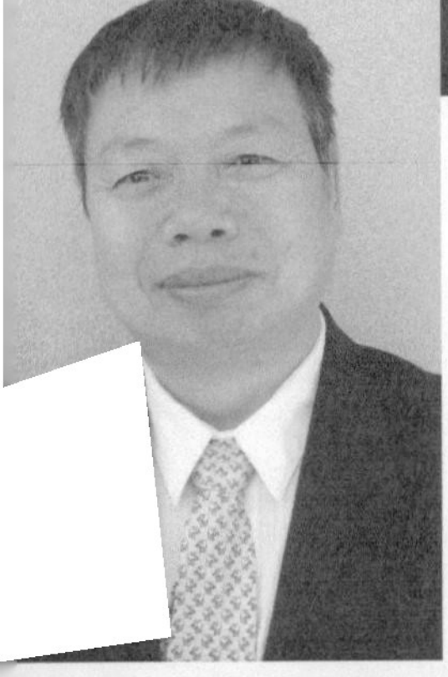
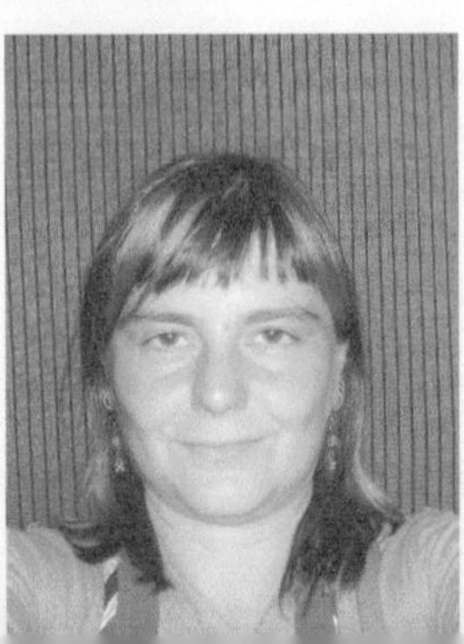

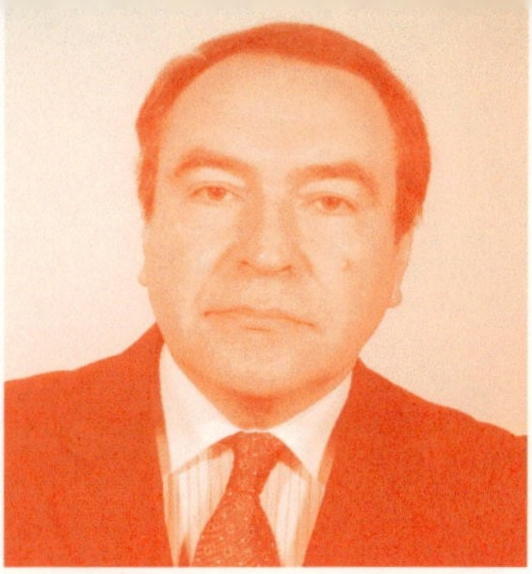

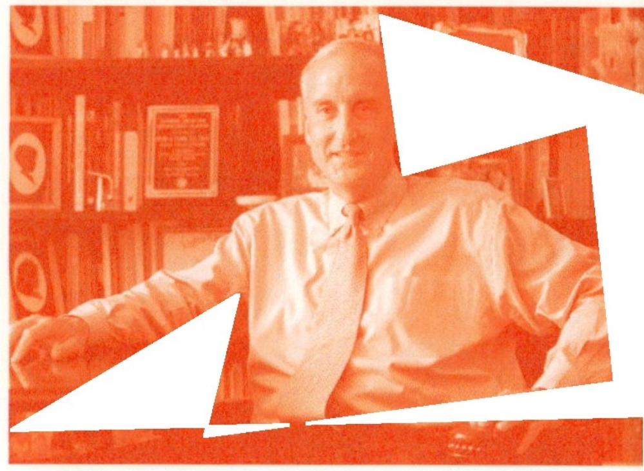

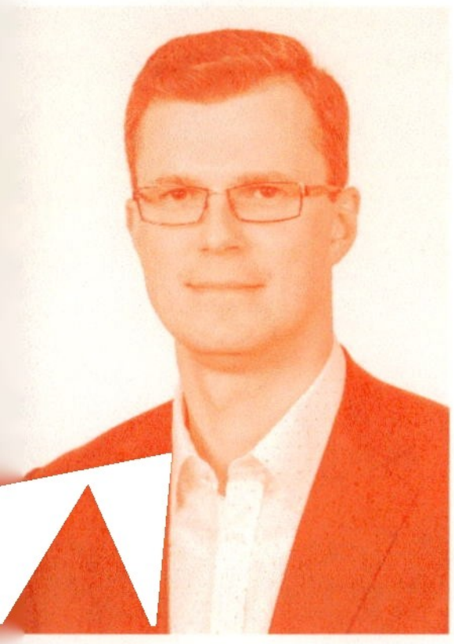

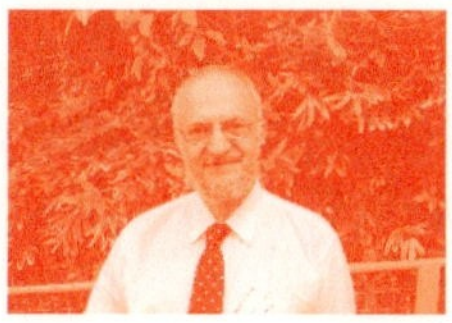

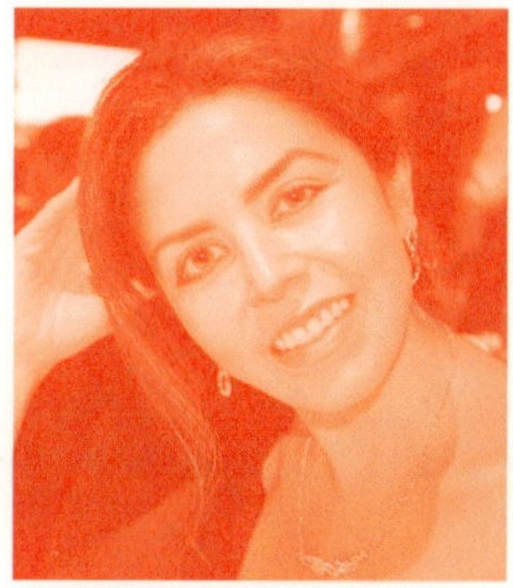

Supporting open minds since 2005

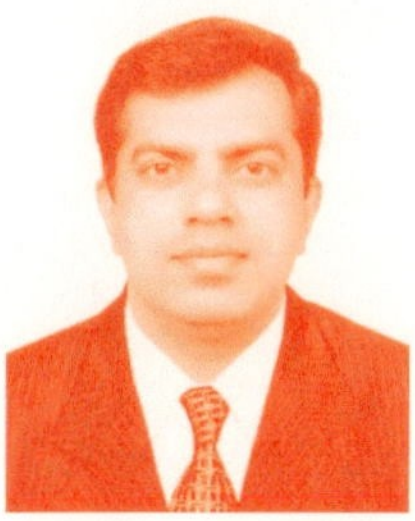

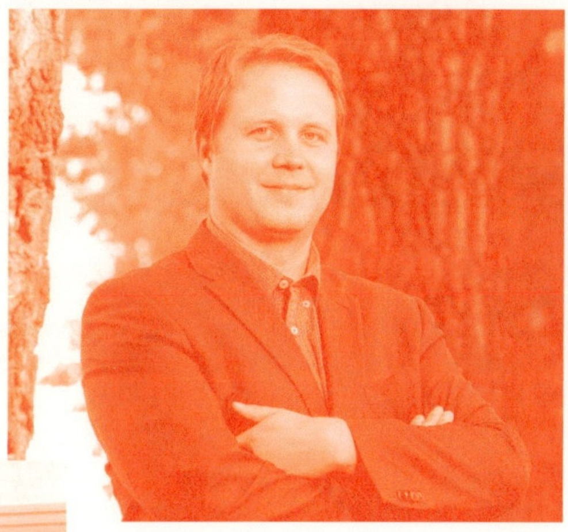

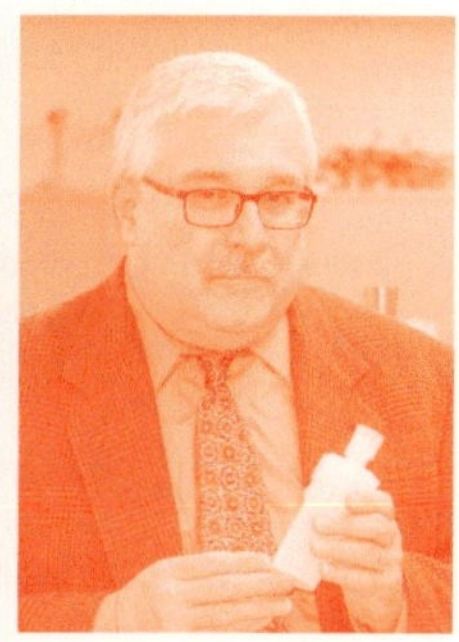

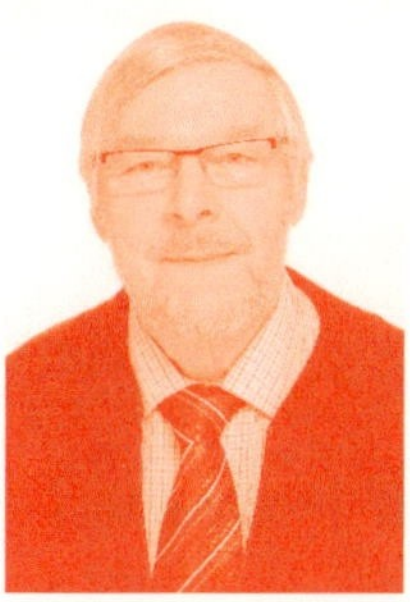

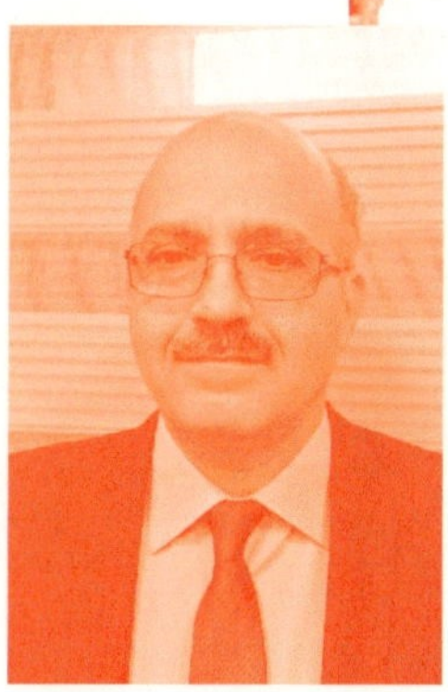

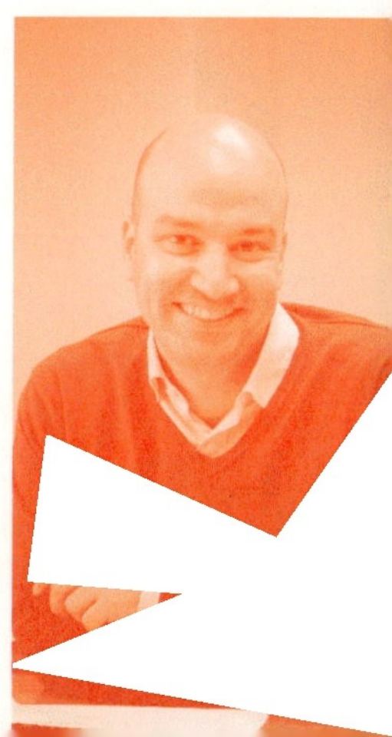

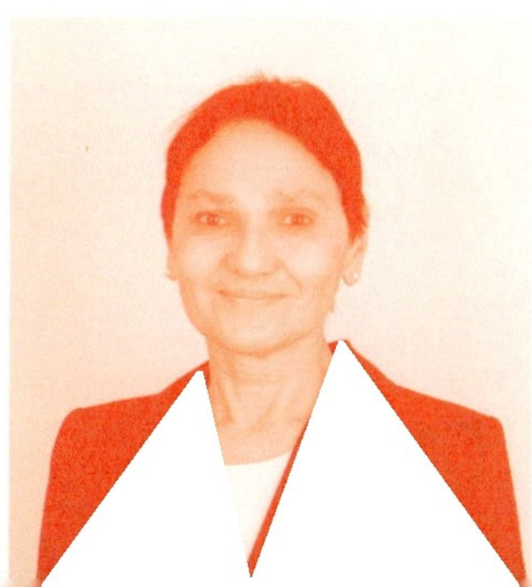

Knowledges on Thyroid Cancer
http://dx.doi.org/10.5772/intechopen.77702
Edited by Omer Engin

Contributors
Dana I Stoian, Andreea Borlea, Ioana Mozos, Laura Cotoi, Sinan Binboga, Eyup Gemici, Elif Binboga, Syed Mudassar, Mosin S Khan, Shariq R Masoodi, Khurshid I Andrabi, Manuel Faria, Carla Sobral, Marcelo Magalhaes, Pietro Giorgio Calò, Fabio Medas, Gian Luigi Canu, Enrico Erdas, Maria Deligiorgi, Dimitrios Trafalis, Omer Engin

© The Editor(s) and the Author(s) 2019
The rights of the editor(s) and the author(s) have been asserted in accordance with the Copyright, Designs and Patents Act 1988. All rights to the book as a whole are reserved by INTECHOPEN LIMITED. The book as a whole (compilation) cannot be reproduced, distributed or used for commercial or non-commercial purposes without INTECHOPEN LIMITED's written permission. Enquiries concerning the use of the book should be directed to INTECHOPEN LIMITED rights and permissions department (permissions@intechopen.com).
Violations are liable to prosecution under the governing Copyright Law.

(cc) BY

Individual chapters of this publication are distributed under the terms of the Creative Commons Attribution 3.0 Unported License which permits commercial use, distribution and reproduction of the individual chapters, provided the original author(s) and source publication are appropriately acknowledged. If so indicated, certain images may not be included under the Creative Commons license. In such cases users will need to obtain permission from the license holder to reproduce the material. More details and guidelines concerning content reuse and adaptation can be found at http://www.intechopen.com/copyright-policy.html.

Notice
Statements and opinions expressed in the chapters are these of the individual contributors and not necessarily those of the editors or publisher. No responsibility is accepted for the accuracy of information contained in the published chapters. The publisher assumes no responsibility for any damage or injury to persons or property arising out of the use of any materials, instructions, methods or ideas contained in the book.

First published in London, United Kingdom, 2019 by IntechOpen
IntechOpen is the global imprint of INTECHOPEN LIMITED, registered in England and Wales, registration number: 11086078, The Shard, 25th floor, 32 London Bridge Street
London, SE19SG – United Kingdom
Printed in Croatia

British Library Cataloguing-in-Publication Data
A catalogue record for this book is available from the British Library

Additional hard and PDF copies can be obtained from orders@intechopen.com

Knowledges on Thyroid Cancer
Edited by Omer Engin
p. cm.
Print ISBN 978-1-78923-983-6
Online ISBN 978-1-78923-984-3
eBook (PDF) ISBN 978-1-83881-891-3

For EU product safety concerns:
IN TECH d.o.o., Prolaz Marije Krucifikse Kozulić 3, 51000 Rijeka, Croatia, info@intechopen.com or visit our website at intechopen.com.

We are IntechOpen, the world's leading publisher of Open Access books
Built by scientists, for scientists

4,200+
Open access books available

116,000+
International authors and editors

125M+
Downloads

151
Countries delivered to

Our authors are among the
Top 1%
most cited scientists

12.2%
Contributors from top 500 universities

CLARIVATE ANALYTICS BOOK CITATION INDEX INDEXED

WEB OF SCIENCE™

Selection of our books indexed in the Book Citation Index in Web of Science™ Core Collection (BKCI)

Interested in publishing with us?
Contact book.department@intechopen.com

Numbers displayed above are based on latest data collected.
For more information visit www.intechopen.com

Meet the editor

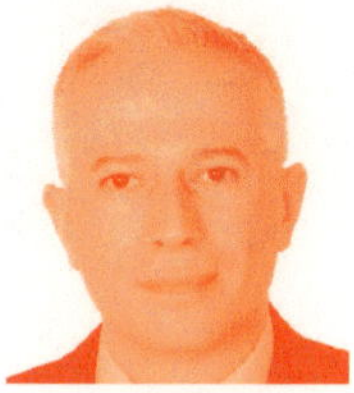

Dr. Omer Engin in an associate professor of general surgery at Health Sciences University, Tepecik Training and Research Hospital, Surgery Department, Turkey. He has published a number of international articles, chapters, and congress papers, and has served as book editor for international published books and as an organizing committee member in a number of international conferences. He is an organization scientific committee member in the International Medical Society Scientific Committee and Athens Institute for Education and Research. He serves as an editorial board member and as a reviewer for many international medical and surgical scientific journals. His specializations are: endocrine surgery, hepatobiliary surgery, bariatric surgery, gastrointestinal surgery, and oncologic surgery.

Contents

Preface

Thyroid cancer is being increasingly diagnosed nowadays. This situation has attracted the attention of scientists and physicians alike. This updated book deals with various aspects of thyroid cancer and has been written by various international authors who have devoted many long and meticulous hours to the subject.

Omer Engin
Izmir Tepecik Eğitim ve Araştırma Hastanesi,
Turkey

Chapter 1

Introductory Chapter: Knowledges on Thyroid Cancer

Omer Engin

1. Introduction

The thyroid gland is located in the neck in front of the trachea. The gland has right and left lobes. The lobes are connected by isthmus. The superior thyroid artery arises from the external carotid artery; inferior thyroid arteries arise from thyrocervical trunks [1].

Superior and middle veins of the thyroid gland drain into the internal jugular vein; the inferior vein of the gland drains into the brachiocephalic vein or directly into the superior vena cava [2, 3].

Superior and inferior laryngeal nerves are important in thyroid surgery.

The superior laryngeal nerve divides into external and internal branches. The external branch stimulates the cricothyroid muscle, so when the nerve is injured, the vocal cord tension is decreased on the side of injury. The internal branch provides sensor innervation to supraglottic and glottic larynx [4, 5].

Another name for the inferior laryngeal nerve is the recurrent laryngeal nerve (RLN). RLN has internal and external branches. The internal branch of RLN supplies sensation of the vocal cords and subglottic areas. The external branch of this nerve sends motor fibres to the intrinsic laryngeal muscles except the cricothyroid muscle. These two nerves may be lacerated in thyroidectomy operations [6].

Thyroid cancer is one of the surgeries often performed in surgical practice. Among thyroidectomy indications, thyroid cancer has an important place. There are significant differences between thyroidectomy due to benign diseases and thyroidectomy due to malignant disease. Complications are also different as the surgical method is different. Oncological rules apply in thyroid cancer surgery. Therefore, the complication rates may be different.

The symptoms of thyroid cancer may be silent as well as may be noticeable. Thyroid cancer can follow a quiet and slow clinical process. Or thyroid cancer can follow a rapid clinical process. Thyroid cancer may be associated with other clinical diseases. Care should be taken in such cases and thyroid cancer should not be overlooked. In general, a palpable nodule is palpated in the neck. Sometimes cervical pathologic lymphadenopathy is palpated or is found on ultrasonographic examination incidentally. In this situation, ultrasound-guided fine needle aspiration biopsy may be needed for histologic diagnosis in the preoperative stage. Thyroid malignancies may progress from the neck into the thorax, so intrathoracic goitre may develop. In general intrathoracic goitre is operated in the neck, but sometimes sternotomy may be needed [7, 8].

Hoarseness can be a sign of thyroid cancer. If the tumour invades the recurrent laryngeal nerve, the vocal cord is paralysed. For diagnosis, thyroid ultrasonography and indirect laryngoscopy may be used [9].

There are noninvasive and invasive methods in the diagnosis of thyroid cancer. Ultrasound-guided fine needle aspiration biopsy can be used as an invasive method. Ultrasonography, one of the noninvasive methods, has been increasingly used in the

IntechOpen

diagnosis of thyroid cancer. Ultrasonography, scintigraphy, computerised tomography, magnetic resonance imaging and PET CT can be used for evaluation of the thyroid cancer and metastases. Preoperative evaluation with imaging tests gives us a route for therapeutic modalities [10, 11].

In thyroid cancer cases, a very good thyroid anatomy should be known. It is very important not to damage the anatomical structures during neck dissection. The anatomy of the thyroid and neck should be well known for a good surgical outcome.

Papillary thyroid cancer is the most common type in the thyroid cancers. Others are follicular thyroid cancer, medullary thyroid carcinomas, anaplastic thyroid carcinomas, primary thyroid lymphomas and primary thyroid sarcomas. Last two malignancies are seen rarely. Hurthle cell cancer is often accepted as a variant of follicular thyroid cancer. Thyroid cancer may have metastasis at the time of diagnosis [12, 13].

Nowadays, various technological innovations have been developed to reduce complications during thyroidectomy. Intraoperative nerve monitoring is one of these innovations. The nerve damage was reduced during thyroidectomy with the nerve monitoring. Do not forget that surgical skills are not an important thing for the prevention of nerve injury. Methylene blue dyeing is another method for identifying of the recurrent nerve. Methylene blue may be given intraarterially or by directly spraying on the tissue [14, 15].

In the thyroidectomy operation, different complications can occur such as hemorrhagia, recurrent nerve injury, trachea laceration, oesophageal laceration, etc. It is important that, if these complications are diagnosed in intraoperative or perioperative time, they may be corrected. For example, if the recurrent nerve is lacerated and is diagnosed by the surgeon, the surgeon can suture the lacerated nerve. But if the injured nerve is diagnosed in the postoperative period, nerve suturing cannot be used. So careful surgical dissection is most important for the prevention of the complications [16, 17]. Another important complication is oesophageal laceration. If the lacerated oesophagus is not diagnosed in the intraoperative period, this can lead to cervical sepsis. When esophagus is lacerated in the operation, intraoperative suturing can be performed intraoperatively. If esophageal laceration is minimal and it can not be recognized intraoperatively, endoscopic endoclips may be choosen as an alternative method [18].

In our book, the issues have been examined by the international elite authors. Our book is not a text book where each subject is processed, respectively. Information about thyroid cancer is given from different perspectives with the original approach.

I hope that our book will be useful to all physicians who are interested in the thyroid.

With my love and respect.

Author details

Omer Engin
Izmir Tepecik Eğitim ve Araştırma Hastanesi, Turkey

*Address all correspondence to: omerengin@hotmail.com

IntechOpen

© 2019 The Author(s). Licensee IntechOpen. This chapter is distributed under the terms of the Creative Commons Attribution License (http://creativecommons.org/licenses/by/3.0), which permits unrestricted use, distribution, and reproduction in any medium, provided the original work is properly cited.

References

[1] Miller FR. Surgical anatomy of the thyroid and parathyroid glands. Otolaryngologic Clinics of North America. 2003;**36**(1):1-7

[2] Maceroni P. Ultrasound features of thyroid, parathyroid, neck lymph nodes: Normal and pathologic pattern. In: Mini mally Invasive Therapies for Endocrine Neck Diseases. Cham: Springer; 2016. pp. 3-13

[3] Sawant DA, Moore TF, Cashell AW. A cadaveric case report of dual thyroid: Ectopic and normal location thyroid with brief review of literature. International Journal of Endocrinology and Metabolism. 2018;**6**(3):201-206

[4] Sun S-Q, Chang RWH. The superior laryngeal nerve loop and its surgical implications. Surgical and Radiologic Anatomy. 1991;**13**(3):175-180

[5] Marchese-Ragona R, Restivo DA, Mylonakis I, et al. The superior laryngeal nerve injury of a famous soprano, Amelita Galli-Curci. Acta Otorhinolaryngologica Italica. 2013;**33**(1):67-71

[6] Ardito G et al. Revisited anatomy of the recurrent laryngeal nerves. The American Journal of Surgery. 2004;**187**(2):249-253

[7] Viola D et al. Prophylactic central compartment lymph node dissection in papillary thyroid carcinoma: Clinical implications derived from the first prospective randomized controlled single institution study. The Journal of Clinical Endocrinology & Metabolism. 2015;**100**(4):1316-1324

[8] Rolighed L, Rønning H, Christiansen P. Sternotomy for substernal goiter: Retrospective study of 52 operations. Langenbeck's Archives of Surgery. 2015;**400**(3):301-306

[9] Jin J. Screening for thyroid cancer. JAMA. 2017;**317**(18):1920-1920

[10] Tajiri K et al. Can ultrasound alone predict papillary thyroid carcinoma with desmoid-type fibromatosis? A retrospective analysis of 13 cases, focusing on the stromal area. Ultrasound International Open. 2018;**4**(02):E39-E44

[11] Vrachimis A et al. [18 F] FDG PET/CT outperforms [18 F] FDG PET/MRI in differentiated thyroid cancer. European Journal of Nuclear Medicine and Molecular Imaging. 2016;**43**(2):212-220

[12] Agrawal N et al. Integrated genomic characterization of papillary thyroid carcinoma. Cell. 2014;**159**(3):676-690

[13] Kam BL et al. Treatment of patients with hurtle cell thyroid carcinoma using [Lu-177-DOTA0, Tyr3] octreotate. Journal of Nuclear Medicine. 2016;**57**(supplement 2):208-208

[14] Lv B, Zhang B, Zeng Q-D. Total endoscopic thyroidectomy with intraoperative laryngeal nerve monitoring. International Journal of Endocrinology. 2016;**2016**:5. http://dx.doi.org/10.1155/2016/7381792 Article ID: 7381792

[15] Sari S, Erhan A, Muslumanoglu M et al. Safe thyroidectomy with intraoperative methylene blue spraying. Thyroid Research. 2012;**5**(1):15. https://doi.org/10.1186/1756-6614-5-15

[16] Muheremu A, AO Q. Past, present, and future of nerve conduits in the treatment of peripheral nerve injury. BioMed Research International. 2015;**2015**:6. http://dx.doi.org/10.1155/2015/237507 Article ID: 237507

[17] Erovic BM, Lercher P. Sural nerve grafting. In: Manual of Head and Neck Reconstruction Using Regional and Free Flaps. Vienna: Springer; 2015. pp. 63-65

[18] Young CA et al. CT features of esophageal emergencies. Radiographics. 2008;**28**(6):1541-1553

Chapter 2

Thyroid Anatomy

Sinan Binboga, Eyup Gemici and Elif Binboga

Abstract

In ancient times, the Celsius first identified the masses in the neck and reported that their surgical removal was fatal. The sources related to thyroid surgery show that the success of the neck masses with the surgical intervention was limited until the second half of the nineteenth century. Among the names leading the development of thyroid surgery in contemporary times are Emil Theodor Kocher, Theodor Billroth, William James Mayo, and William Stewart Halsted. In this chapter, we will be investigating thyroid gland embryology, histology, and anatomy that is essential to the practicing thyroid surgeon.

Keywords: thyroid gland, anatomy, embryology, histology, vascularization

1. Introduction

This chapter will discuss the thyroid anatomy including macroscopic/microscopic structure, thyroid embryology, and also vascular composition and innervation. The nuclear medicine imaging, ultrasound, and biopsy of the thyroid in the evaluation of nodules and differentiation of benign from malignant disease have a very precious place. Generally, the neck is the part of the body that separates the head from the torso. The midline in front of the neck has a prominence of the thyroid cartilage termed the laryngeal prominence. Between the laryngeal prominence and the chin, the hyoid bone can be felt; below the thyroid cartilage, a further ring that can be felt in the midline is the cricoid cartilage. Between the cricoid cartilage and the suprasternal notch, the trachea and isthmus of the thyroid gland can be felt. The quadrangular area is on the side of the neck and is bounded superiorly by the lower border of the body of the mandible and the mastoid process, inferiorly by the clavicle, anteriorly by a midline in front of the neck, and posteriorly by the trapezius muscle. The main arteries in the neck are the common carotids, and the main veins of the neck that return the blood from the head and face are the external and internal jugular veins. The thyroid is located in front of the neck between the levels of the C5 and T1, joined by the isthmus, bridging to the trachea. The basic anatomy is best appreciated in **Figure 1**. The size and shape of the thyroid lobes vary widely in normal patients. The shape of lateral lobes is longitudinally elongated in tall subjects, whereas in shorter subjects, the gland is more oval. In the newborn the thyroid gland is approximately 19 mm, with an anteroposterior (AP) diameter of 8–9 mm. By 1 year of age, the mean length is 25 mm with 12–15 mm AP, whereas the mean length is approximately 40–60 mm, with mean 13–18 mm AP in adults. The thyroid gland is slightly larger and heavier in women. It shows a little more growth in pregnancy and menstruation [1–4]. The thyroid gland is an organ of the endocrine system that maintains body metabolism, growth, and development through the synthesis, storage, and secretion of thyroid hormones. These hormones include

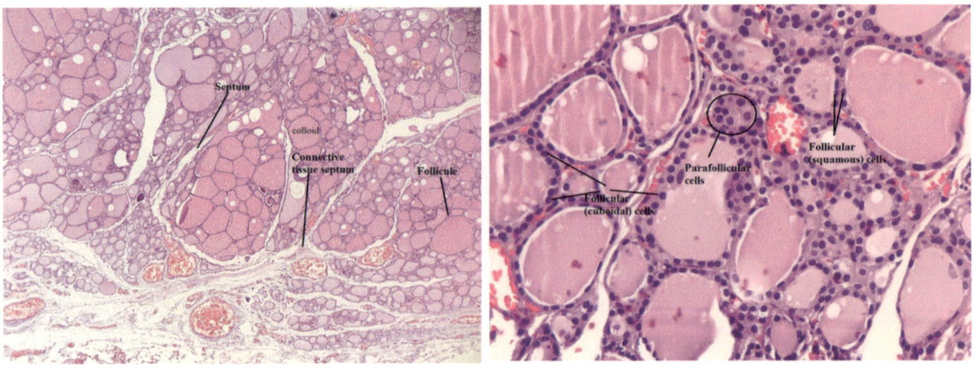

(a) (b)

Figure 1.
a) General thyroid gland histology including fibrous capsule,septum, follicules and reticular fiber meshwork
b) Thyroid gland cell types; parafollicular and follicular cells

triiodothyronine (T3), thyroxine (T4), and calcitonin. Food-energy metabolism of cells is stimulated by T3 and T4. Calcitonin has a minor role in regulation of calcium levels. Disorders of the thyroid may result from thyroid gland dysfunction, which is regulated by the pituitary and hypothalamus glands. An appreciation of the embryological development of the thyroid and parathyroid glands facilitates comprehension of some of the various anatomical and pathological processes. The worldwide guides of various associations such as the American Thyroid Association (ATA), American Association of Clinical Endocrinologists (AACE), American College of Endocrinology (ACE), and Associazione Medici Endocrinologi (AME) are used in the evaluation of the pathological processes [5].

2. Embryology of the thyroid gland

The primordial thyroid gland is one the earliest endocrine organs. It is detectable during the starting day 24 in the embryo. Throughout the 4th to 7th weeks of gestation, it slowly migrates to the final location. It is developed from pharyngeal endoderm cells and derived from the foramen caecum in the tongue base and also connected to the tongue base via thyroglossal duct until week 10. It consists of two lobes, and both lobes (lobus dexter and lobus sinister) are connected together with isthmus. There is a small lobe known as "the pyramidal lobe" mostly derived from the left lobe of the thyroid and attached to the hyoid bone. Calcitonin-secreting parafollicular thyroid ("C") cells are derived from a combination of cells migrating from the neural crest and a fifth pharyngeal pouch structure [5, 6].

There are clinically relevant various pathologic consequences of this embryogenesis, for example, hypothyroidism, thyroglossal duct cyst, medullary carcinoma, and fistulas.

3. Histology of the thyroid gland

The thyroid gland is a unique endocrine gland with follicles and extracellular components storing large amounts of hormone in an inactive form [7]. The gland is enveloped by a fibrous capsule, and a fine collagenous septum divides the thyroid gland into lobules consisting of numerous thyroid follicles which are closely packed ring-shaped structures with an average diameter of about 200 μm [8]. The follicles are embedded within the meshwork of reticular fibers (**Figure 1a**) [9].

The thyroid follicles are the main functional and structural components of the gland which synthesize and release T3 and T4 in the center of follicles. Each follicle is filled with colloid, which is a gelatinous substance containing the stored form of T3 and T4. In active glands, the colloid is predominantly basophilic, whereas in inactive glands, it is acidophilic. In highly activated glands, this colloid is not only reduced in amount but also shows vacuoles [9].

There are types of thyroid cells, i.e., follicular cells and parafollicular cells. The follicular or principal cells are responsible for T3 and T4 production. These cells are usually simple cuboidal cells but may change to simple squamous (inactive) or columnar cells (active) depending on their states of secretion (**Figure 1b**). H&E staining of thyroid gland shows that the follicular cells have basophilic cytoplasm and a round nucleus with one or more distinct nucleoli. Golgi apparatus is located in the supranuclear position. Ultrastructurally, the cells contain the organelles showing both secretory and absorptive characteristics and short microvilli on the apical surface of cells. In basal location, cells contain a large number of rough endoplasmic reticulum. In apical location, cells contain small vesicles morphologically related to Golgi apparatus and a large number of endocytotic vesicles lysosomes defined as colloidal resorption droplets [10].

Parafollicular or clear cells (C cells) are the second type of thyroid cells, located within the follicular epithelium or as small clumps adjacent to the follicles. These cells are relatively large oval or ellipsoid cells with round nuclei and pale cytoplasm and are found lying on the basal follicular membrane. These cells have an extensive unstained cytoplasm often difficult to distinguish in H&E sections and therefore called “C” cells [7]. These cells produce calcitonin hormone released in response to high blood calcium and inhibits the activity of the osteoclasts [11].

4. Macroscopic anatomy of the thyroid gland

The thyroid gland is enveloped by the fascia consisting of the anterior and posterior parts of the deep cervical fascia. The gland weighs approximately 10–20 g, and each lobe measures an average of 5 cm in length, 2.5 cm in width, and 1.5 cm in depth [12]. The gland is slightly heavier and bigger in size during menstruation and pregnancy [13]. Thyroid lobes are located lateral to the trachea and esophagus, anteromedial to the carotid sheath, and posteromedial to the strap muscles (sternohyoid, sternothyroid, and superior belly of the omohyoid) and are innervated by the ansa cervicalis (ansa hypoglossi), overlying from the level of the fifth cervical vertebra down to the first thoracic vertebra (**Figure 2a**) [13, 14]. The shape of the gland varies from an H to a U form, consisted of two elongated lateral lobes with superior and inferior poles that are joined at the midline by an isthmus. The length of the isthmus is in between 12 and 15 high, connecting the two lobes. Occasionally, the isthmus may be absent, and the gland exists as two separate lobes (**Figure 2b**).

A pyramidal lobe presents in approximately 50% of patients extending toward the hyoid bone, to which it may be attached by a fibrous or fibromuscular band [14]. The most lateral extension of the thyroid lobes is the Zuckerkandl tubercles (ZTs). These tubercles are condensed thyroid parenchyma located in the cricothyroid junction, at the junction point of the medial thyroid with the ultimobranchial bodies, and have an important vicinity with the recurrent laryngeal nerve (RLN). ZTs develop from the embryologic fusion of the ultimobranchial body with the median anlage and the lateral thyroid anlages of the fourth pharyngeal pouch. The dissection of this tissue is important because the RLN is located below the ZTs located in the posterolateral of the thyroid gland [15, 16].

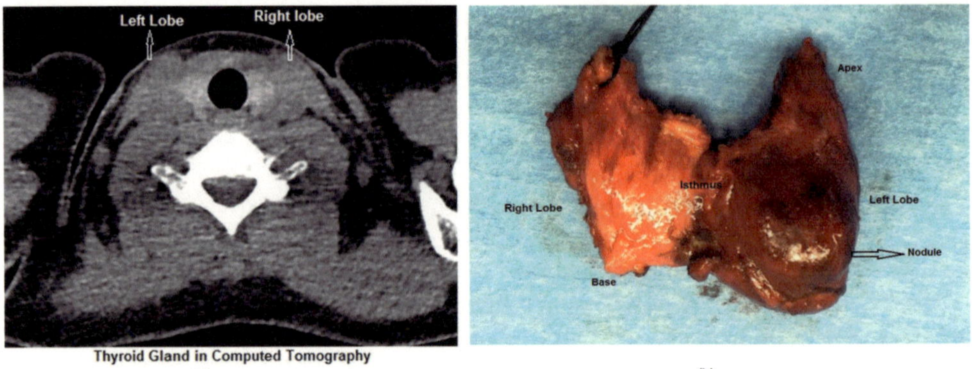

(a) (b)

Figure 2.
a) Thyroid gland in computed tomography b) Macroscopic anatomy of the thyroid gland

Thyroglossal duct extends along the path of thyroid descending from the foramen cecum at the base of the tongue to the lower neck. The cysts of this duct are the most commonly encountered congenital cervical anomalies in humans. They are usually asymptomatic but occasionally become infected by oral bacteria. The carcinomas of the duct are extremely rare, and approximately 1–2% of are found to be cancer, which are usually papillary carcinomas (85%) [12, 17, 18].

A thin layer of the front and back of the deep cervical fascia wraps the thyroid lobes. This fascia joins the capsule by two suspensory ligaments, namely, the anterior and posterior suspensory ligaments. The anterior suspensory ligament extends from the superior medial aspect of each thyroid lobe to the cricoid and thyroid cartilage. The posterior ligament, known as the Berry ligament, connects the thyroid to the cricoid cartilage and upper rings of the trachea. The ligament of Berry is closely attached to the cricoid cartilage and has important surgical implications due to its connection to the RLN. The RLN usually enters deep into the posterior suspensory ligament [14]. During the retracting of the thyroid gland on the medial side, it should not be compelling, because it may cause RLN to be stretched and injured. In addition, rupture of the vena thyroidea media may occur bleeding. Care should be taken not to cause nerve damage during the dissection and hemostasis to control bleeding. There are two superior and two inferior parathyroid glands. The parathyroid glands are small structures adjacent to or occasionally embedded in the thyroid gland. Usually, two pairs of parathyroid glands lie in proximity to the thyroid gland. The inferior glands migrate further and have more chance of being in ectopic sites [19, 20].

5. Microscopic anatomy of the thyroid gland

The thyroid gland is a highly vascular organ, among other endocrine organs, in a sense that there is a rich blood flow with large amounts of anastomosis in the gland. Arterial supply is bilateral from both the external carotid system and superior thyroid artery and subclavian system with the lower thyroid branch of the thyrocervical trunk. It may be a single thyroid ima artery arising from the brachiocephalic artery [21].

The superior thyroid arteries originate from the ipsilateral external carotid arteries and are divided into anterior and posterior branches in the apex of the thyroid lobes. Inferior thyroid arteries originate from the thyrocervical shortly after the origin of the subclavian arteries. The inferior thyroid arteries extend from the neck to the back of the carotid sheath and enter the thyroid lobes at the midpoints. Thyroidea ima, the arteries born directly from the aorta or innominate, enters the isthmus or replaces a missing lower thyroid artery in 1–4% of individuals. The inferior thyroid artery passes through the recurrent laryngeal nerve (RLN) and requires the identification of RLN before the arterial branches are ligated. The inferior thyroid artery provides an arterial supply of the cervical esophagus with subclavian artery and branches directly from the aorta, intercostal arteries, and tracheobronchial arteries [22].

There are three main venous pathways of the thyroid: superior, middle, and inferior thyroid veins. The superior thyroid vein accompanies the superior thyroid artery and drains to the internal jugular vein but not accompanied by the middle thyroid vein. There are several inferior thyroid vessels that frequently flow into the internal jugular or brachycephalic veins [12].

5.1 Innervation of the thyroid

RLN is a branch of the vagus nerve, responsible from the laryngeal motor function and feeling. The left RLN is looped from the vagus nerve to the back of the aorta, and the right RLN revolves around the right subclavian artery. During thyroidectomy, since these nerves rise along the trachea near the thyroid gland, the surgeon should pay attention to protect them. The inferior thyroid artery and its terminal branches are closely related to the RLN at the entrance point of the thyroid gland. Sometimes, the nerve can be confused with a branch of the artery. Compared to the artery, it is less regular, rounded, and elastic [23]. A small, red, curved vein called vasa nervorum is usually seen in the wall of the nerve. The left RLN rises straight along the tracheoesophageal groove, while the right RLN is more inclined and lateral than the left one. However, numerous variations have been defined, so care should be taken in every case. In the two upper tracheal rings, the RLN is embedded at the back of the suspensory ligament, called the Berry ligament. This ligament extends to backward of the recurrent nerve and tightly connects the thyroid to the trachea and esophagus. At this point, there is a posterior artery near the recurrent nerve, which gives a small branch to the thyroid gland and is not easy to be attached to this artery (**Figure 3**) [23, 24].

The superior laryngeal nerve is also a branch of the vagus nerve. On the pharynx side, the internal carotid descends from the back of the artery and is divided into

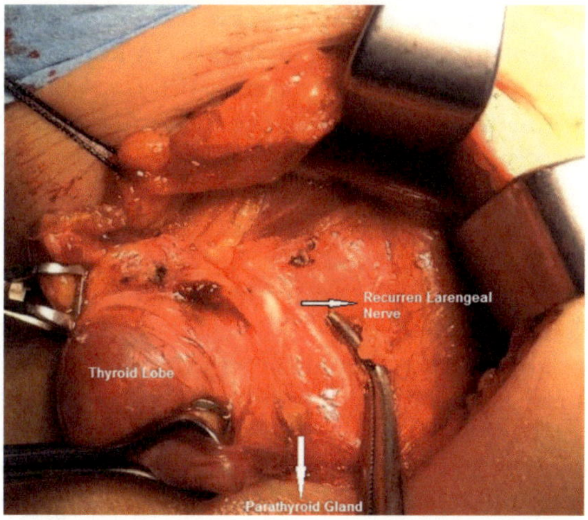

Figure 3.
Thyrid gland location with nerve and parathyroid gland

two arms: the external laryngeal nerve as the motor nerve and the internal laryngeal nerve as the sensory nerve. The superior laryngeal nerve contributes to the pitch of voice, and its paralysis can lead to significant contraction of pitch range, vocal fold vibratory phase asymmetry, and acoustic aperiodicity, thus leading to an overall poor vocal quality [24]. There is a close relationship between the superior thyroid artery and the external branch of the superior laryngeal nerve. This nerve injury may cause high-pitched noises. In order to prevent damage to the external branch of the superior laryngeal nerve, it is recommended to ligate the superior thyroid arteries as low as possible during thyroidectomy. The cricothyroid artery, a branch of the superior thyroid artery, is located in the cephalic portion of the upper pole and moves toward the midline on the cricothyroid ligament. This vessel may be damaged during cricothyroidotomy and may cause bleeding. Care should be taken in large area hemostasis to control bleeding. Ligating the veins one by one prevents nerve damage. Classification of the external branch of the superior laryngeal nerve according to the risk of potential damage [12] is given below.

Type 1: The nerve crosses the superior thyroid vessels more than 1 cm above the border of the thyroid upper pole.

Type 2a: The nerve crosses the vessels less than 1 cm above the border of the thyroid upper pole.

Type 2b: The nerve crosses the vessel below the border of the thyroid upper pole.

The recurrent laryngeal nerve (on the right, after exiting the superior thoracic cavity) may be located in the neck root, in the lateral carotid artery, in the medial trachea, and in the triangle formed by the superior thyroid lobe.

The right recurrent laryngeal nerve usually enters the larynx at an angle of 0–30° in the tracheoesophageal groove. In the left recurrent laryngeal nerve, this angle is about 15–45°. Recurrent laryngeal nerve passes through the posterior of the inferior thyroid artery in 61% of cases, anterior in 32%, and the branches of the artery in 7% of cases. The lower parathyroid glands are located proximal to the inferior laryngeal nerve, and the upper parathyroid glands are located distal to the nerve. Recurrent laryngeal nerve is found in 60–70% of cases in the tracheoesophageal groove, 20–25% in the lateral of the trachea, and 5% in the posterior of the trachea.

In 35–80% of cases, RLS is divided into branches before entering the larynx. Typically, extralaryngeal branching is in two forms as motor and sensory branch. However, two to eight extralaryngeal branches have been described in the literature. Its linear extension and its light yellow color make it known macroscopically.

The right inferior laryngeal nerve is 32 cm long, and the left is approximately 43 cm long. Since the left inferior laryngeal nerve has a longer course in the tracheoesophageal groove, the majority of nerve injuries occur in this side.

Nonrecurrent laryngeal nerve was reported in 0.3–0.8% of cases. Nonrecurrent laryngeal nerve exits the cervical section of the vagus at the level of the larynx or thyroid gland and directly enters the larynx at the level of the cricothyroid joint without forming a loop [25].

The intraoperative methylene blue spraying technique could be used in thyroid surgery. Methylene blue will be sprayed over the thyroid lobe and perilober area. Tissues, especially parathyroides, the recurrent laryngeal nerve, and the inferior thyroid artery could be evaluated [26].

Recurrent nerve damage after thyroid surgery varies between 0 and 11%. Complications are more frequently seen in subtotal thyroidectomies and secondary surgeries than total thyroidectomies and primary surgeries, whereas they are inversely correlated with surgeon experience. Posterior cricoarytenoid muscle palpation without electromyography provided that follow-up of glottic pressure applications and peroperative observation of vocal folds. However, the fact that the practice is both difficult and does not give very healthy results is an important limitation of this method. Postoperative complications were reduced, and surgical duration was significantly reduced by the use of peroperative recurrent nerve monitoring. Measurements are made with surface electrodes integrated in endotracheal intubation tubes. The device alerts the surgeon with sound. In addition, the current changes in the device screen can be recorded and provide legal basis for the surgeon [27].

In patients undergoing peroperative recurrent nerve monitoring, selection of anesthesia is important.

The continued effect of the muscle relaxant agent will affect the results completely. Intubation can be done without using any muscle relaxant. And also, it can be done with using agents which effect in a short time and break down in a short time. For this purpose, succinylcholine is often preferred as a short-acting depolarizing neuromuscular blocking agent [28].

If there is a nerve injury, different methods of recurrent nerve repair, such as microsuturing gluing and grafting, have been proposed [29]. Direct microsuture is preferable when the defect is no longer than 5 mm and the primary repair can be completed without tension [30]. After transection of RLN, immediate reconstruction could be performed by a direct, "end-to-end" anastomosis of neural stamps, by three to four perineural stitches of 7-0 nylon thread, using microsurgical instruments [31]. Cyanoacrylate glue has also been proposed for nerve repair but has been criticized for its toxicity, excessively slow resorption, and risk of inflammatory reaction in the perineural tissues [32].

When the proximal stump of the RLN cannot be used, grafting should be done using the transverse cervical nerve, supraclavicular nerve, or ansa cervicalis [33]. First, start to identify ansa cervicalis on the surface of the internal jugular vein, and branches to the sternothyroid muscles could be dissected. The proximal end of the major branch could anastomosed to the distal RLN stump [34].

5.2 Lymphatics of the thyroid

The lymphatic drainage of the thyroid gland is wide and flows in a versatile pattern. The Hollinshead pattern of drainage is divided into four different ways as the median superior drainage, median inferior drainage, right/left lateral drainage, and posterior drainage [35].

The median superior drainage passes through three to six lymphatic vessels originating from the upper edge of the isthmus and the upper middle edge of the lateral lobes. These lymphatic veins move upward in the direction of the larynx and end in the digastric nodes. Some of the lymphatics can flow into one or two (Delphian) nodes in the throat immediately above the isthmus [23]. Secondarily, the anterior tracheal nodes under the thyroid through the lymphatic channels move downward from the upper jugular nodes on either side of the neck or from the Delphian nodes to the frontal side of the thyroid gland [12, 36].

The median inferior drainage consists of several lymphatic vessels draining to the inferior portion of the isthmus and the lower medial parts of the lateral lobes [36, 37]. These lymphatic channels follow the inferior thyroid veins to terminate before the tracheal and brachycephalic nodes [12, 13]. Right and left lateral drainage patterns originate from the lymphatic bodies at the lateral border of each lobe [12, 25]. The superior thyroid artery and vein are ascended, followed by the lower thyroid artery at the bottom [13, 36]. Between these two groups, the lymphatic ducts move lateral, anterior, or posterior to the carotid sheath to reach the lymph nodes of the internal jugular vein [12–14, 36]. In rare cases, these lymphatic vessels drain directly into the subclavian vein, jugular vein, or thoracic duct without flowing to the lymph node [38].

The posterior drainage pattern begins in the lymphatic vessels draining to the inferomedial parts of the lateral lobes to discharge into the lymph nodes along the RLN track [12, 36]. Rarely, a lymphatic body that rises posteriorly to the upper part of the lobe reaches to the retropharyngeal nodes [36].

Several models of lymphatic drainage of the thyroid gland have been proposed, and all of them are true and comprehended from the same basis. Another simplified drainage model is that emergency lymphatic drainage enters the periglandular nodes, followed by the preterminal and paratracheal nodes along with the RLN and then to the mediastinal lymph nodes [14, 36].

Although lymph node metastasis is known to increase recurrence, its effect on prognosis and survival is still being discussed [39, 40]. All patients with lateral LN recurrence could be therapeutic neck dissection and RAI ablation therapy as adjuvant treatment [41].

Author details

Sinan Binboga[1*], Eyup Gemici[2] and Elif Binboga[3]

1 General Surgery Department, Alsancak Nevvar Salih Isgoren Hospital, Izmir, Turkey

2 Bakirkoy Dr.Sadi Konuk Training and Research Hospital, Istanbul, Turkey

3 Faculty of Medicine, Department of Intensive Care, Dokuz Eylul University, Izmir, Turkey

*Address all correspondence to: dr.binboga@hotmail.com

IntechOpen

© 2019 The Author(s). Licensee IntechOpen. This chapter is distributed under the terms of the Creative Commons Attribution License (http://creativecommons.org/licenses/by/3.0), which permits unrestricted use, distribution, and reproduction in any medium, provided the original work is properly cited.

References

[1] Gray H. Anatomy of the Human Body. Philadelphia: Lea & Febiger, 1918; 2000

[2] Hoyes AD, Kershaw DR. Anatomy and development of the thyroid gland. Ear, Nose, & Throat Journal. 1985;**64**(10):318-332

[3] Lai SY, Mandel SJ, Weber RS. Chapter 119: Management of thyroid neoplasms. In: Cummings Otolaryngology: Head and Neck Surgery. 4th ed. Philadelphia: Mosby; 2005. pp. 2687-2718

[4] Ahuja AT, Antonio GE, editors. Diagnostic and Surgical Imaging Anatomy: Ultrasound. Manitoba, Canada: Amirsys; 2007

[5] Arrangoiz R, Cordera F, Caba D, Muñoz M, Moreno E, León EL. Comprehensive review of thyroid embryology, anatomy, histology, and physiology for surgeons. International Journal of Otolaryngology and Head & Neck Surgery. 2018;**7**(4): 160-188. DOI: 10.4236/ijohns.2018.74019

[6] Dominique Dorion Thyroid Anatomy. Available from: https://reference.medscape.com/article/835535-overview

[7] Young B, Heath JW. Wheater's Functional Histology. 4th ed. Edinburg: Churchill-Livingstone; 2000. pp. 315-317

[8] Singh I. Human Embryology. 6th ed. India: Jaypee Brothers Medical Publishers; 2005. pp. 119-123

[9] Cui D. Endocrin system. In: Atlas of Histology with Functional and Clinical Correlations. First ed. Baltimore: Lippincott Williams & Wilkins, a Wolters Kluwer business; 2011. pp. 325-334

[10] Ross MH, Pawlina W. Endocrine organs. In: Histology: A Text and Atlas, with Correlated Cell and Molecular Biology. 6th ed. Baltimore: Lippincott Williams & Wilkins, a Wolters Kluwer business; 2010. p. 755

[11] Lokanadham S, Subhadra Devi V. Thyroid Gland—Morphology & Histogenesis. Germany: LAP LAMBERT Academic Publishing; 2013. pp. 20-21

[12] Skandalakis JE. Neck: Thyroid gland. In: Skandalakis JE, editor. Surgical Anatomy. The Embryologic and Anatomic Basis of Modern Surgery. 14th ed. Vol. 1. Athens: Paschalidis Medical Publications; 2004

[13] Cummings CW. Thyroid anatomy. In: Cummings CW, editor. Head and Neck Surgery. 3rd ed. St. Louis: Mosby; 1998

[14] Williams PL, Bannister LH. Thyroid gland. In: Gray's Anatomy. 38th ed. New York: Churchill Livingstone; 1995

[15] Sheahan P, Murphy MS. Thyroid tubercle of Zuckerkandl: Importance in thyroid surgery. Laryngoscope. 2011;**121**(11):23357. DOI: 10.1002/lary.22188PMid:21898449

[16] Costanzo M, Caruso LA, Veroux M, et al. The lobe of Zuckerkandl: An important sign of recurrent laryngeal nerve. Annali Italiani di Chirurgia. 2005;**76**(4):337-340. PMID: 16550870

[17] Plaza CP, Lopez ME, Carrasco CE, Meseguer LM, Perucho Ade L. Management of well-differentiated thyroglossal remnant thyroid carcinoma: Time to close the debate? Report of five new cases and proposal of a definitive algorithm for treatment. Annals of Surgical Oncology. 2006;**13**:745-752

[18] Doshi SV, Cruz RM, Hilsinger RL Jr. Thyroglossal duct carcinoma: A large case series. The Annals of

Otology, Rhinology, and Laryngology. 2001;**110**:734-738

[19] Fancy T, Gallagher D, Hornig JD. Surgical anatomy of the thyroid and parathyroid glands. Otolaryngologic Clinics of North America. 2010;**43**: 221-227. DOI: 10.1016/j.otc.2010.01.001

[20] Akerström G, Malmaeus J, Bergström R. Surgical anatomy of human parathyroid glands. Surgery. 1984;**95**:14

[21] Toni R, Della Casa C, et al. Anthropological variations in the anatomy of the human thyroid arteries. Thyroid. 2003;**13**:183-192

[22] Lal G, Clark OH. Thyroid, parathyroid, and adrenal. In: Schwartz Principles of Surgery. 10th ed. pp. 1523-1524

[23] Orestes MI, Chhetri DK. Superior laryngeal nerve injury: Effects, clinical findings, prognosis, and management options. Current Opinion in Otolaryngology & Head and Neck Surgery. 2014;**22**(6):439-443

[24] Youn YK, Lee KE, Choi JY. Color Atlas of Thyroid Surgery. South Korea: Springer Heidelberg; 2014. pp. 5-6

[25] Miller FR. Surgical anatomy of the thyroid and parathyroid glands. Otolaryngologic Clinics of North America. 2003;**36**:1-7

[26] Tian W, Jiang Y, Gao B, Zhang X, Zhang S, Zhao J, et al. Application of nano-carbon in lymph node dissection for thyroid cancer and protection of parathyroid glands. Medical Science Monitor. 2014;**20**:1925-1930

[27] Dralle H, Sekulla C, Lorenz K, Brauckhoff M, Machens A, the German IONM Study Group. Intraoperative monitoring of the recurrent laryngeal nerve in the thyroid surgery. World Journal of Surgery. 2008;**32**:1358-1366

[28] Chu KS, Wu SH, Lu IC, et al. Feasibility of intraoperative neuromonitoring during thyroid surgery after administration of nondepolarizing neuromuscular blocking agents. World Journal of Surgery. 2009;**33**:1408-1413

[29] Miyauchi A, Inoue H, Tomoda C, et al. Improvement in phonation after reconstruction of the recurrent laryngeal nerve in patients with thyroid cancer invading the nerve. Surgery. 2009;**146**:1056-1062

[30] Sanuki T, Yumoto E, Minoda R, et al. The role of immediate recurrent laryngeal nerve reconstruction for thyroid cancer surgery. Journal of Oncology. 2010;**2010**:846235

[31] Dzodic R, Markovic I, Santrac N, et al. Recurrent laryngeal nerve liberations and reconstructions: A single institution experience. World Journal of Surgery. 2016;**40**:644-651

[32] Choi BH, Kim BY, Huh JY, et al. Microneural anastomosis using cyanoacrylate adhesives. International Journal of Oral and Maxillofacial Surgery. 2004;**33**:777-780

[33] Gurrado A, Pasculli A, Pezzolla A, et al. A method to repair the recurrent laryngeal nerve during thyroidectomy. Canadian Journal of Surgery. 2018; **61**(4):278-282

[34] Miyauchi A, Masuoka H, Tomoda C, et al. Laryngeal approach to the recurrent laryngeal nerve involved by thyroid cancer at the ligament of Berry. Surgery. 2012;**152**:57-60

[35] Zollinger R et al. Atlas of Surgical Operations. 9th ed. New York: McGraw-Hill; 2010

[36] Hollinshead WH. Anatomy for Surgeons. 3rd ed. Vol. 1. Philadelphia: Lippincott Williams and Wilkins; 1982

[37] Larsen WJ. Human Embryology. 3th ed. Philadelphia: Churchill Livingstone; 2011. pp. 372-374

[38] Stephen C, Munnoch DA. Lymphoedema of the upper limb: A rare complication of thyroid surgery? BML Case Reports. 2016;**2016**. DOI: 10.1136/bcr-2016-214376

[39] Mazefferi EL, Jhiang SM. Long term impact of initial surgical and medical therapy on papillary and folliculary thyroid cancer. The American Journal of Medicine. 1994;**97**:418-428

[40] Yamashita, H, Noguchi S, Murakami N, Kawamoto H, Watanabe S. Extracapsular invasion of lymph node metastasis is an indicator distant metastasis and poor prognosis in patients with thyroid papillary carcinoma.Cancer. Dec 15 1997;**80**(12):2268-72

[41] Lim YC, Liu L, Chang JW, Koo BS. Lateral lymph node recurrence after total thyroidectomy and central neck dissection in patients with papillary thyroid cancer without clinical evidence of lateral neck metastasis. Oral Oncology. 2016;**62**:109-113

Chapter 3

Advanced Ultrasound Techniques in Preoperative Diagnostic of Thyroid Cancers

Andreea Borlea, Laura Cotoi, Ioana Mozos and Dana Stoian

Abstract

The most precise evaluation of thyroid masses is by high-sensitive ultrasound. Complementary to B-mode ultrasound, elastography can add valuable information by determining tissue stiffness—an important predictor for malignancy. All major guidelines recommend nodules with high suspicious ultrasound characteristics larger than 1 cm to be addressed to ultrasound-guided fine needle aspiration biopsy (FNAB) to rule out malignancy. The main limitation of this procedure is represented by indeterminate cytology, which accounts for up to 20–25% of biopsy results. Molecular markers imply elevated costs and their performance needs further study. Elastography may be helpful in establishing the optimal therapeutic attitude for this cytological category. Currently, there are two ultrasound elastography methods available for assessing tissue stiffness using the parallel deformation to the applied force direction (strain) or the perpendicular deformation to the force direction (shear wave). These methods will be presented and compared in this chapter, with their indications and limitations for a better understanding of their application in nodular thyroid pathology.

Keywords: thyroid cancer, ultrasound, elastography, strain, shear wave, malignancy risk assessment

1. Introduction

Thyroid cancer incidence increased in the last three decades by up to 211%, not only as a result of a better ability to detect very small lesions, by means of high-resolution ultrasonography, but also secondary to a real increase of thyroid cancer incidence, regardless of size, gender, or age groups [1, 2]. Even in these conditions, the prevalence of thyroid cancer, in the entire group of thyroid nodules, reaches a percentage of 15% [3], the main challenge for clinicians being the correct identification of which nodules to refer to fine needle aspiration cytology (FNAC) or directly to surgery, and which to follow by means of ultrasound evaluation [2, 4].

"A thyroid nodule is defined as a discrete lesion within the thyroid gland that is ultrasonographically distinct from the surrounding thyroid parenchyma" [4]. Nodules are usually noticed either by the patient when causing clinical disturbances or compressive symptoms, or by the clinician when performing a thyroid screening or a radiologic procedure such as carotid ultrasound or computed tomography of the neck [5].

When evaluating a thyroid nodule, first line step is represented by running laboratory tests (thyroid-stimulating hormone and thyroid hormones) and performing ultrasound evaluation of the gland. Evaluation goals include identification of the small percentage of malignant nodules, of those that impair thyroid function and of compressive symptoms (dysphonia and dyspnea) [6, 7].

Personal or family history of thyroid cancer, significant exposure to radiations, increases the malignancy risk of the nodule and should be screened for [8].

It is desired to have uniform and standardized reports, given the increased accessibility of the ultrasound equipment and considerable number of clinicians that perform this type of evaluation. Reports will always record nodule position, number, extracapsular relations, and the following features of the lesions: size, shape, margins, echogenicity, echo texture, internal composition (solid, cystic, or mixed), presence of calcifications, and vascular pattern [2].

There are some US features described that are considered highly specific for malignancy, as the presence of microcalcifications, rim calcifications, infiltrative margins, extrathyroidal extension, mostly solid composition, marked hypoechoic texture, and "taller than wide" shape, respectively, the vertical diameter bigger than the transverse diameter. Spongiform appearance, smooth margins, and cystic composition are associated with benignity [6].

Vascularization assessment is considered to have poor interobserver agreement and it has highly dependent on the US equipment used [9].

Additionally, abnormal cervical lymph nodes should be assessed, especially in patients with intermediate- and high-risk thyroid nodules [10].

Various authors and societies proposed risk-stratification systems for thyroid nodules on US. They were initially introduced by classifying thyroid nodules which displayed any suspicious feature as malignant. Thus, starting with Kim et al. in 2002, risk-stratification systems were conceived as qualitative grading systems.

Assessment based on a combination of US features has been proposed as a better method of risk stratification. The system developed into a quantitative scoring system, on which the concept of thyroid imaging reporting and data system (TI-RADS) is based. Horvath et al., inspired by the previously existing breast imaging reporting and data system (BI-RADS) score, introduced it in 2009. Since then, the concept has permanently developed; each new concept proposed having its advantages and limitations regarding their practical application [11]. There are also data suggesting TI-RADS quantification is better than individual assessment of the US characteristics [12].

Different diagnostic qualities are described for each model: Park model: Se = 82%, Sp = 65% [13]; Kwak model: Se = 97.4%, Sp = 29.3% [14, 15].

Diagnostic accuracy for Russ' TI-RADS model was evaluated comparatively on gray scale alone and associated with elastography score. When compared to cytological results, the study showed Se = 95.7, Sp = 61%, and NPV = 99.7% for gray scale only; Se = 98.5%, Sp = 44.7%, and NPV = 99.8% for the combined model using gray scale + elastography. For the operated group, these models were also compared to pathology results showing Se = 93.2% for gray-scale TI-RADS and Se = 96.7% for gray scale + elastography. It was estimated that the number of nodules sent to FNAB decreased by 33.8% [9, 10, 16].

Stoian model also calculated strain ratio for each nodule, apart from qualitative SE scoring, with excellent diagnostic value (AUC = 0.95761, 95% confidence interval (CI)). In this case, Se = 97.93%, Sp = 86.20%, and NPV = 97.26%. Nodules required for FNAB decreased by 43.7% [17].

The 2017 ACR–TIRADS applied on 100 thyroid nodules showed an overall Se = 92% and Sp = 44%, with a 29% reduction in the number of nodules that require biopsy [18].

US-guided FNAB represents the next step in thyroid nodule evaluation and is considered to be the most accurate and cost-efficient preoperative method for identifying malignancy in thyroid nodular lesions, but its indications are broad and differ in the guidelines [19, 20]. Complications are rare and are usually represented by local pain or minor hematomas, but patients are still sometimes reluctant to undergo this procedure [21]. Prior the FNAB, the patients can be questioned for the use of blood thinner drugs and hematologic disease such as bleeding-clotting disorders.

A category-based reporting system was developed and standardized for thyroid FNAB specimens by The Bethesda System for Reporting Thyroid Cytopathology (and it has been broadly adopted). Based on this reporting system, thyroid nodule cytology can be classified in one of the following six categories: (I) nondiagnostic, (II) benign, (III) atypia or follicular lesion of undetermined significance (AUS or FLUS), (IV) (suspicion of) follicular neoplasm, (V) suspicious for malignancy, and (VI) malignant [22–24].

Each category has its evidence-based recommendation for further clinical behavior according to its estimated malignancy risk. The real challenge concerns the management of indeterminate cytology lesions (Bethesda categories III–V) [22].

Benign cytology accounts for 60–70% of FNAs, malignant findings for about 5%—papillary thyroid carcinoma (PTC) being the most common, and indeterminate cytology for 10–20% of specimens—atypical modifications, follicular or Hurthle cell cancers. The indeterminate category has anywhere from 15 to 60% risk of malignancy, depending on the specifics of the report. Studies recently showed that molecular markers can help future distinction between benign and malignant nodules in this cytological category but there are no recommendations currently in use [20].

The American Association of Clinical Endocrinology 2016 guidelines recommend FNAB for nodules with high US risk if they are ≥10 mm, for intermediate US risk nodules ≥20 mm, and low US risk lesions >20 mm that are increasing in size or have thyroid cancer history. For nodules between 5 and 10 mm in diameter with high-risk US characteristics, they recommend FNAC or watchful waiting. Functioning nodules on scintigraphy that lack suspicious US characteristics do not have recommendation for FNAC [4].

The American Thyroid Association (ATA) Management Guidelines refer to FNAC also for intermediate risk nodules >10 mm [19].

The Korean Thyroid Association (KTA) 2016 Revised Guideline recommends that highly suspicious nodules <1 cm should undergo FNAC in order to avoid unnecessary long-term follow-up, given that 20–40% of nodules in this category are benign [25].

The number of nodules addressed to FNAC could be reduced, as 60–80% of FNACs reveal benign lesions; this low percentage of malignancy detected in the nodules sent to FNAC based on US imaging criteria points out the real need for a more accurate US diagnostic evaluation [4, 6].

There are some drawbacks regarding FNAC results. About 5% of cases are considered qualitative or quantitative insufficient for diagnostic, and Bethesda III and IV categories are inconclusive for a final treatment recommendation. In the presence of indeterminate cytology, the clinical judgment relies again on patient background (clinical risk categories) and ultrasonography aspect [22, 26].

2. Ultrasound elastography—nodule stiffness as a malignancy risk-stratification parameter

US elastography noninvasively evaluates the stiffness of a thyroid nodule by measuring the distortion that appears when the nodule is compressed by external pressure (strain elastography) or by assessing the attenuation of the shear waves (shear-wave elastography) generated by the transducer [10].

Elasticity is the ability of tissue to resist deformation when an external force is applied, or to resume its original shape after the force is removed [27]. Loss of elasticity of a tissue on palpation or elastography ("virtual palpation") generates suspicion of malignancy. Most solid tumors are mechanically different from adjacent tissues, presenting increased stiffness (decreased elasticity) owing to desmoplastic transformation—more collagen and myofibroblasts [27, 28].

There are some fibrous benign tumors that can be hard on elastography (histiocytofibromas) and some malignant nodules with nonmodified elasticity that can be missed by elastography (follicular carcinomas) [28, 29].

The different US elastography techniques that are currently available carry various limitations in relation to the tissue shear properties and they may be in some cases complementary [30]. Elastography can be easily used in the evaluation of the thyroid gland considering its conveniently superficial location, but it is still not widely adopted in practice or included in all the risk-stratification systems [31].

Presently, only one thyroid US elastography guideline has been published—the "European Federation of Societies for Ultrasound in Medicine and Biology (EFSUMB) Guidelines and Recommendations." Recommendations are in favor of using elastography as an extra tool to gray-scale ultrasound and for the follow-up of nodules formerly benign in FNAB [32].

2.1 Strain (quasistatic) elastography

Strain elastography (SE) was the first to be used and most implemented technique on US systems. Usually, very slight external pressure is applied by the operator (or by acoustic radiation force impulse (ARFI)), or more recently, it has the sensitivity to detect minimal endogenous physiological motion (vascular beam movements and muscle contraction) [28, 30]. The imaging methods are a little different for each manufacturer so each equipment will display images with slightly different characteristics [33].

SE equipment does not offer direct quantification of stress. Elastograms illustrate relative stiffness and are calculated from the signal differences previously and after compression, being displayed in parallel with B-mode image (split-screen) or overlaid on the conventional B-mode image. Stiffness of the tissue is displayed usually in a continuous color map from red (soft or no strain) to green (intermediate or equal strain) to blue (hard or no strain). There are some systems available on the market that use a reverse color scale [34, 35].

A visual colorimetric analysis based on the displayed qualitative map image will be made [32]. Two scoring systems have been proposed for the qualitative assessment of nodule elasticity: the Asteria and Rago systems. Asteria classifies nodules on a scale from 1 (entirely elastic nodule) to 4 (entirely stiff nodule). Rago includes the first four Asteria classes with the addition of the fifth score (entirely stiff nodule, infiltrating in the posterior shadowing area) [35]. Lesions that appear homogenous or with low stiffness are considered benign, while lesions that present increased stiffness are considered to have high malignancy risk [28].

SE machines use special software for an objective semiquantitative determination providing a numeric value: *the strain ratio* (*SR*). This method of elasticity assessment represents the ratio between strain value in the neighboring thyroid parenchyma and the mean nodule strain (parenchyma-to-nodule ratio) or between the strain in a neighboring strap muscle and the thyroid nodule (muscle-to-nodule ratio) [32]. Probability of cancer grows with a higher strain ratio [35]. A study conducted by Aydin et al. in 2014 showed that there are no significant differences between muscle-to-nodule ratio and parenchyma-to-nodule ratio, suggesting that the first ratio could be safely used instead of last ratio in evaluating malignancy risk when the thyroid parenchyma is abnormal [36]. SR is considered to be more accurate than qualitative elasticity assessment. The final value will represent the average of three measurements [37].

Widely different cutoff values have been described for the SR (between 1 and 5), currently there is no general agreement: ≥ 2 (Se = 97.3%, Sp = 91.7%) [38]; ≥ 2.09 (Se = 90.6%; Sp = 93%) [39]; ≥ 2.73 (Se = 89.3%; Sp = 73.2%) [40]; and ≥ 3.79 (Se = 97.8%; Sp = 85.7%) [41]. Most of these studies included only solid nodules.

Elastography imaging to B-mode size ratio (EI/B ratio) has been suggested to be useful in evaluation of breast lesions [42].

The area ratio (AR) is a semiquantitative assessment for SE in virtual touch equipment that compares the nodule area on virtual touch image and B-mode, calculating the mean of the three most accurate measurements. A malignancy cutoff of 1.08 was suggested [43].

Hard area ratio is the ratio between the nodule hard area and the whole nodule area. Different cutoff values for malignancy have been proposed: ≥ 0.45 (Se = 98.2%; Sp =81.2%) [40] and ≥0.6 (Se = 92.9%, Sp = 91.3%). This parameter is highly dependent on the examiner and has poor reproducibility [37].

The elasticity contrast index is available on Samsung machines and measures the strain oscillation within a nodule and then uses complex calculation to determine local contrast. In a malignant lesion, there are large differences between low and high strain regions, inducing important local contrast [44].

When choosing the place of the ROI, some aspects have to be taken into consideration. It should be as proximal to the transducer as possible, it should cover the entire nodule and "as much of the adjacent parenchyma as possible." Manual compression is quantified on most of the machines for better reproducibility: optimal compression in Hitachi machines is considered between 3 and 4 and > 50 in Siemens machines [32, 37].

There is a huge body of evidence regarding the diagnostic qualities of the SE method in defining benign versus malignant lesion.

In a meta-analysis conducted in 2010 by Bojunga et al. that included eight studies (639 nodules), RTE recognized thyroid malignancy with overall mean Se = 92% (88–96 CI) and mean Sp = 90% (85–95 CI). A significant heterogeneity was found for specificity of the different studies [45].

Rago et al. conducted a study on 195 nodules, which concluded that RTE elastography had Se = 94.9%, Sp =90.3%, PPV = 71.1%, and NPV = 98.6% in predicting malignancy in nodules with indeterminate or nondiagnostic cytology. Worth mentioning is the high NPV of high elasticity-score nodules, which strongly predicts benignity [46].

Another valuable study from Italy evaluated SE diagnostic accuracy on 498 nodules showing Se = 97% and NPV = 97% when at least one suspicious US parameters was also present [47].

A meta-analysis that included 20 studies evaluating SE diagnostic value in benign or malignant nodules showed a pooled Se = 85% (95% CI, 79–90%), Sp = 80% (95% CI, 73–86%), NPV = 97% (95% CI, 94–98%), and PPV = 40% (95% CI, 34–48%) [48].

Some of SE limitations are represented by its subjectivity, operator-dependency, and compressibility-dependency [49].

Increased stiffness can be found in benign nodules with coarse calcification or fibrosis, leading to false-positive results [45, 50].

When the evaluated lesion is located deeper, an elastogram can be obtained if lesion can be visualized in the B-mode image, but it may require application of more stress by the examiner, which could alter the color map for more superficial structures. If nodules are too deep, a false-positive stiff image can appear as a result of reduced stress transmission [32].

Nodule size is not considered to interfere with SE evaluation accuracy, although there are some studies that reported affected performance on nodules larger than 3 cm or very small lesions. WFUMB guidelines consider nodules larger than 3 cm cannot be evaluated correctly because of their deeper parts and lack of healthy adjacent tissue. Coalescent nodules can also not be assessed by SE [32, 37, 51].

Carotid pulsations interfere when external pressure is applied, particularly in transverse incidence, the incidence being preferred for elastography with internal force [32].

The reference surrounding parenchyma in the ROI should have at least 50% green color to obtain an accurate strain ration [37].

Other limitations of SE are presence of peripheral rim calcification—increased stiffness; large cystic component—SE in nodules with cystic components should be assessed only for the solid component; necrosis—can present soft areas; nodules under 5 mm—although a low size limit for SE use was not established; and obese patients [50, 51].

It is clear that strain elastography accuracy is highly dependent on the examiner's training. The interobserver variability has been evaluated by several studies that recently showed excellent agreement between multiple observers [32]. It seems that strain ratio is easily learned compared to elasticity score interpretation [52].

Different pathologies of the thyroid nodules can have an impact on SE appearance. Currently, it is known that follicular carcinomas may appear elastic on SE, so elastography is not a useful tool for evaluating this type of thyroid malignancy (44% false-negative findings). Other particular pathologies that appear soft on elastography and may lead to false-negative results are medullary carcinomas and metastatic carcinomas [32, 45].

2.2 Shear-wave elastography

Shear waves are defined as transverse elements of particle displacement which are very quickly attenuated by the tissue. Shear represents a modification of shape, without a modification of volume [35, 53]. Tissue propagation of shear waves is much slower in comparison to longitudinal waves. They do not propagate well in water, being rapidly attenuated, but they do propagate in elastic media [54].

Shear-wave elastography (SWE) is more operator-independent, and therefore, more reproducible [35]. Quantitative and qualitative assessment of tissue elasticity can be obtained by measuring the shear wave speed. Several applicable methods are available [27].

1D Transient elastography is widely used for estimating liver fibrosis (Fibroscan and Echosens). It cannot be performed with a standard transducer on regular ultrasound equipment. The probe used by this device incorporates an US transducer as well as a vibrating device that exerts an external vibrating "punch" to generate shear waves that will propagate through tissues [27].

In monoplane shear-wave elastography (pSWE), ARFI mechanically excites the tissue in the region of interest (ROI) using acoustic push pulses which generate localized tissue displacements in the US axial direction—perpendicular to the surface. Shear wave speed measurements can be made up to 8 cm in depth (m/s) [14, 30]. This approach is implemented on devices produced by Phillips (ElastPQ) and Siemens (VitualTouch Quantification, VTQ) [27].

Biplane shear-wave elastography (SWE, 2D SWE, 3D SWE) offers a real-time display of a color quantitative elastogram overlaid on a B-mode image and assessment of shear wave speed [27]. Supersonic shear wave uses focused ultrasonic beams that spread through the whole imaging area, displaying on a color map the velocity (m/s) of the shear wave or directly the elasticity (kilopascals) for every pixel in the ROI. A series of parameters in the ROI can be measured: maximum stiffness, mean stiffness, and standard deviation (SD) [35].

The following 2D-SWE technologies are currently available on US machines by: Siemens (Virtual Touch Imaging Quantification, VTIQ), SuperSonic Imagine (SWE), Philips (SWE), Toshiba (Acoustic Structure Quantification), and GE Healthcare (2D-SWE) [27].

The largest recent meta-analysis by Zhang et al. included 16 studies that used ARFI-generated SWE to evaluate 2436 nodules had mean Se = 0.80 (95% CI, 0.73–0.87) and Sp = 0.85 (95% CI, 0.80–0.90) in detecting malignancy. Both Se and Sp were found significantly heterogeneous in all the included studies [55].

Another meta-analysis (Dong et al.) on 13 retro/prospective studies detected high ARFI VTQ efficacy in detecting thyroid cancer, with pooled Se = 86.3% (95% CI, 78.2–91.7) and Sp = 89.5% (95% CI: 83.3–93.6) [56].

A meta-analysis by Lin et al. included 15 studies that used point-SWE or 2D SWE to investigate 1867 nodules. The pooled Se = 84.3% (95% CI, 76.9–89.7%), Sp = 88.4% (95% CI, 84.0–91.7%), PPV = 27.7–44.7%, and NPV = 98.1–99.1% [57].

All the mentioned meta-analyses concluded that SWE (pSWE and 2-D SWE) are useful in detecting thyroid malignancy as a complementary tool to gray-scale US, which is also a stated recommendation of WFUMB 2017 guidelines [32].

Five to ten consecutive measurements are needed in order to obtain a valid median result [32].

Cutoff values again range widely and have been reported for shear-wave velocity between 2.4 and 4.7 m/s [32].

One study on 476 nodules established an EI cutoff mean value of above 85 kPa (Se = 95%) or one maximum value of above 94 kPa [58]. Another study on VTQ of ARFI reported a cutoff point for velocity = 2.87 m/s and for SWV ratio = 1.59. The study also pointed out this SWE method has highest diagnostic value for nodules >20 mm [59].

Other studies reviewed in the WFUMB guidelines showed cutoff values ranging from 2.55 to 2.75 m/s [60–63].

Interobserver and intraobserver reproducibility were reported to be high. One study conducted by Grazhdani et al. showed high concordance rate (k = 0.75) between two observers [64].

For the characterization of the thyroid lesion, a quantitate measurement for the mean value or maximum value of an elasticity is used. Similar to SE, an SR can be obtained by comparing adjacent normal parenchyma or surrounding muscle [32].

Some of ARFI technique limitations will be briefly presented.

The size of the ROI is fixed (5 × 6 mm or 20 × 20 mm)—small nodules cannot be accurately measured. Also for nodules smaller than 20 mm, wave velocity is not stable. Composition of nodules: cystic composition or calcifications cannot be evaluated—it is impossible to place the ROI inside the nodule. Depth is an important limitation for both pSWE and 2D SWE—the ARFI cannot penetrate nodules deeper than 4–5 cm; ARFI can measure velocities only up to 9 m/s—harder nodules or areas will not be evaluated properly: the value "x.xx m/s" will be shown. Nodules that are located on the thyroid isthmus are a challenge due to their interposition between the stiff trachea and the skin [32, 37].

Again, not all malignant nodules are elastic. Follicular carcinomas are described as soft lesions and are difficult to differentiate from benign lesions. A study by Samir et al. proposed a cutoff value of 22.3 kPa for distinguishing thyroid follicular cancer from benign follicular lesions (Se = 82%; Sp = 88%) [65].

For accurate results, an experimented examiner should always perform SWE evaluation of the thyroid. The pressure applied on the transducer can influence the evaluation results [32].

There are also clear recommendations that in the presence of a stiff nodule, the FNAB is recommended, regardless the conventional US characteristics.

In the AACE guidelines, a nodule with high stiffness is directly included in the intermediate risk group, elevated stiffness being listed as one of the AACE criteria for FNAB. There is a grade-B recommendation for nodules that are stiff on elastography to be addressed to FNAB [7].

Also, in the presence of indeterminate cytology findings, they suggest that elastography to be considered for extra information. Combined elastography and B-mode US is presented to be more trustworthy when excluding nodules from biopsy evaluation [7].

ATA guidelines acknowledge usefulness of US elastography for noninvasive assessment of malignancy risk when accurate evaluation can be made, but it can neither recommend its universal adoption, nor its replacement of classic US assessment [19].

European Thyroid Association (ETA) guidelines also state that elastography, with its high NPV, can be a helpful instrument for thyroid nodule evaluation and it may be used together with gray-scale US, but not replace it [10].

2.3 RTE versus SWE elastography

As mentioned in the EFSUMB guidelines and showed in literature data, both SE and SWE represent a useful tool in thyroid nodule stratification of malignancy risk, complementary to gray-scale evaluation [32].

Different studies have reported a wide range of values for Se and Sp when comparing the two-elastographic methods.

A big meta-analysis on 71 studies with a total of 16,624 patients showed that RTE is slightly better in differentiating benignancy from malignancy in thyroid lesions, with pooled Se = 82.9% for RTE; Se = 78.4% for SWE and Sp = 82.8% for RTE; and Sp = 82.4% for SWE [66].

A head-to-head comparison of two elastographic methods was made only in a few studies.

In a publication by Liu et al., 49 patients (64 nodules) underwent both SWE and RTE evaluation and results were compared to pathology results. For SE, qualitative assessment was made using Rago classification (score 4–5 considered as malignancy suspicious) and for SWE—min and max mean elasticity were measured, cutoff mean value was 38.3 kPa, with Sp = 68.4%; Se = 86.7%; NPV = 86.7%; PPV = 68.4% for SWE and Sp = 79%; Se = 84.4%; NPV = 83.3%; PPV = 64.7% for RTE. The study established that SWE is a promising method for the evaluation of thyroid malignancy risk, with similar value to RTE, its sensitivity being a little lower and its specificity a little higher [67].

A 2017 meta-analysis (Hu et al.) is evaluating 22 studies, which simultaneously evaluated diagnostic performance for thyroid malignancy using both RTE and SWE techniques. The results showed that the pooled Se = 0.79 (95% CI, 0.73–0.84), Sp = 0.87 (95% CI, 0.79–0.92) for SWE compared with Se = 0.84 (95% CI, 0.76–0.90), Sp = 0.90 (95% CI, 0.85–0.94) for RTE, was significant lower for SWE technique ($p < 0.05$) [49].

Another study evaluated 138 nodules using gray-scale US, ARFI imaging and qualitative strain elastography. Combination of ARFI and RTE specificity for detecting malignancy increased by 20% (Sp = 92 vs. 72% for RTE only), but sensitivity decreased by 28% (Se = 48 vs. 76% for RTE alone). When ARFI cutoff was adapted for the combined methods (ES 3–4 and ARFI ≥1.11 m/s), sensitivity was unchanged, specificity increased by just 3%. Therefore, there was no significant change in accuracy of finding malignant nodules when combining the two methods [63].

Although most literature data suggest RTE is slightly more powerful in differentiating thyroid cancer, there is currently no consensus about which method is better and both SE and SWE proved to add important value to classic US evaluation in the preoperative approach of thyroid nodules.

2.4 Elastography: place in indeterminate cytology results

Nondiagnostic and indeterminate cytology represent the great limitations of FNAC and gray-scale US can sometimes be poorly predictive. About half of these nodules can avoid surgery by performing a second biopsy [68]. There was one study that reported higher prevalence of cancer on repeat FNAB, maybe as a consequence of the class of high-risk nodules that underwent second FNAB [69].

For the clearance of this cytological category, there is currently a general proposal to use molecular markers, but there is still no consensus regarding which panel should be used [70].

Several molecular markers have been studied in indeterminate FNAB cytology findings. The most studied mutations/rearrangements include BRAF, RAS, RET/PTC, and PAX8/PPARγ. These markers can predict ("rule in") malignancy with very high sensitivity, having a high positive predictive value (PPV) but if they are not present, malignancy cannot be "ruled out," having a low sensitivity and negative predictive value (NPV) [70, 71].

The most common molecular tests used in this rapidly developing field will be shortly presented. The Afirma Gene Expression Classifier (GEC) is a microarray test which investigates mRNA expression of 167 genes [72]. This test has been reported to have high NPV (up to 95%) in the Bethesda III and IV categories, but low PPV (14–57%), which makes it useful only as a "rule-out" test [72, 73]. ThyGenX test identifies over 100 mutations associated with thyroid cancer, using a next-generation-sequencing (NGS). ThyraMIR is a newer test (used complementary to the ThyGenX) that analyzes 10 different microRNA molecules that are considered to contribute to cell differentiation and proliferation in thyroid pathology. Combining ThyGenX and ThyraMIR in nodules with indeterminate cytology showed Se = 89%, Sp = 85%, NPV = 94%, and PPV = 74% [72, 74]. ThyroSeq v2 includes analysis of a panel of >1000 mutations and RNA alterations, with Se = 90%, Sp = 93%, PPV = 83%, and NPV = 96%, suggesting that this test may be useful as both "rule-in" and "rule-out" test for Bethesda III and IV cytology [72, 75]. It has been suggested that the thyrotropin receptor (TSHR) mRNA test can be useful in indeterminate nodules, its expression being helpful for early diagnosis of PTC [72, 76, 77].

Currently, there is no individual molecular marker that can certainly rule out malignancy in indeterminate nodules and it is still debatable if there is a cost-effective combination of these markers that can be used [4, 70, 71].

Elastography has been suggested to define more accurately the presurgical malignancy risk in this cytological category to help clinician's decision whether to repeat biopsy or follow-up [32].

A study by Rago et al. tried to refine diagnosis in this category of nodules (142 indeterminate and 53 nondiagnostic). All patients have been examined by gray-scale US, color Doppler, and qualitative RTE (modified Ueno score). Indeterminate cytology score 1—highly elastic nodule—was found strongly predictive of benignity ($p < 0.0001$); combination of scores 2 and 3 showed Se = 96.8%, Sp = 91.8%, and NPV = 99.0% for predicting malignancy. In nondiagnostic cases, Sp, Se, and NPV showed poorer Se, Sp, and NPV for all elastography scores. When considering both indeterminate and nondiagnostic, the overall Se = 94.9%, Sp = 90.3%, and NPV = 91.3% for scores 2 and 3 [46].

In another study, qualitative RTE failed to make a correct distinction between benignity and malignancy in thyroid nodules, cancer was found in 50% of nodules scored 1 or 2 on elastogram and in 34% of score 3 nodules. Quantitative assessment of elasticity was suggested [78].

A comparison between 2D-SWE (VTIQ) and molecular testing (Afirma GEC) was made in a prospective study in nodules with indeterminate FNAC. SWV cutoff for malignancy risk was defined at above 3.59 m/s with Se = 83.9% and Sp = 79.2%. SWV measurements were made in the stiffest section; authors mention that measurements of a larger area may result in a decreased SWV. The GEC-suspicious group had Se = 90.3% and Sp = 74.2% (PPV of only 47.5%, but NPV of 96.7%). The study concluded that both SWV and GEC can independently predict thyroid cancer with similar diagnostic value and are particularly useful in this cytological category [79].

A more complex study compared diagnostic efficiency of SWE, semiquantitative SE (strain index), classic US, CEUS, and BRAF mutation test in indeterminate cytology, but the number of evaluated nodules was relatively small. The study outcomes confirmed a slightly better efficiency for RTE compared to SWE in distinguishing malignancy; strain index was the one parameter that showed significant correlation with pathology results. RTE and SWE do not seem interchangeable but may be used complementary. Interestingly, when strain index, SWV, and BRAF mutation were considered together, Sp was enhanced, but Se was lower compared to US findings alone [68].

This cytological category still remains uncertain in diagnosis, and in some cases, a strategy that combines advanced ultrasound methods was documented to provide higher accuracy in diagnosis than use of a single technique [68]. More studies are required concerning this approach.

2.5 Contrast-enhanced ultrasound (CEUS)

The use of contrast agents in ultrasonography has widely expanded in clinical use and may play an important role in identifying thyroid cancers by evaluating tumor microcirculation. New-generation contrast agents (SonoVue) are administered intravenously and contain sulfur hexafluoride microbubbles that stay in the blood flow for a while. The examiner focuses the US image on the ROI and a contrast-enhanced image is displayed, detecting microvascular changes in the lesion that classic Doppler cannot display [80].

CEUS has already changed approach in management of liver lesions, significantly improving the number of unnecessary biopsy indications [81].

In studies where CEUS was performed on thyroid lesions, malignity was indicated by hypoenhancement and heterogeneity [80]. Hypoenhancement can be explained by the absence of blood supply in the central area of the tumor, due to thrombus formation, vascular compression, and necrosis. Neovascularization is mainly marginal, promoting tumor expansion [82]. Heterogeneity is explained by the complex and aberrant composition of cancerous lesions (fibrotic, presence of calcifications, and necrosis areas) [80, 82].

Other indicators of malignancy are the time of wash-in and wash-out, but results are controversial. Some studies described early wash-in and wash-out in malignant lesions [83, 84], while others have shown late-phase enhancement for thyroid cancers compared to perinodular tissue [85] or no significant difference in the time of enhancement for benign versus malignant nodules [86].

Adenomas are characterized by homogeneity and peripheral ring enhancement [80].

Two recent meta-analyses on CEUS diagnostic accuracy showed the pooled Se = 0.88 (95% CI, 0.85–0.91); pooled Sp = 0.90 (95% CI, 0.88–0.92) [87]; and a pooled Se = 0.853, pooled Sp = 0.87 [88].

Some benign nodules showed pattern described for malignant ones and vice versa, so an assessment of both elastography and CEUS was combined in some articles.

A study by Zhan et al. aimed to evaluate the aid of CEUS in diagnosis of thyroid malignancy. First, 200 thyroid nodules were evaluated using ARFI technique. A number of 40 nodules that were in the "gray zone" underwent CEUS. ARFI accurately diagnosed 82% of the total nodules, while CEUS accuracy was 90% ($p < 0.05$) [89].

Cantisani et al. compared Q-elastography with CEUS in thyroid cancer assessment. Study results showed that both methods outclassed gray-scale US, but Q-elastography was more sensitive than CEUS (Se = 95%, Sp = 88% for Q-elastography; Se = 79%, Sp = 91% for CEUS) [83].

However, more studies are required for evaluating the true usefulness of this relatively new and promising technique in the differentiation of malignant from benign thyroid nodules.

3. Conclusions

Given the great number of thyroid lesions and the rising incidence of thyroid cancer, a correct preoperative distinction between benignity and malignancy in nodular pathology is crucial.

Ultrasound elastography represents the most important advance in US imaging since Doppler. It proved to serve as an important tool in selecting candidates for surgery. Elastography is a noninvasive, nonirradiating method that can be easily learned, adds only a few minutes to classic US evaluation, but provides truly valuable additional information. Unfortunately, this technique is still quite new and not widely used in clinical practice, so its universal adoption cannot be recommended by the guidelines, but there is important evidence of its clinical utility and its application in current practice is increasing. As any imaging technique, it holds its limitations [90].

This technique cannot replace the classic, gray-scale ultrasound, and should be used complementary to it [7, 10, 25].

Due to its high NPV, thyroid nodules that are scored soft on elastography are highly likely to be noncancerous and can be followed-up, avoiding FNAB [91]. Therefore, elastography reduces the need for FNA by up to 43% of cases compared to gray-scale risk stratification [17]. It also identifies stiff nodules that need biopsy and can be missed by gray-scale US alone. Even lesions with low-risk features, but high stiffness, are recommended for FNAB [91].

In the case of indeterminate cytology, clinical judgment can be a real challenge for practitioners. Elastography proved to predict malignancy better than B-mode parameters and can be essential in further management decision for nodules in this category.

For an accurate result, it is important that the evaluation should be performed by an experienced operator.

Conflict of interest

There is no conflict of interest.

Abbreviations

FNAB	fine needle biopsy
US	ultrasonography conventional
Se	sensitivity
Sp	specificity
NPV	negative predictive value
PPV	positive predictive value
AACE	American Association of Clinical Endocrinology
ATA	American Thyroid Association
ETA	European Thyroid Association
EFSUMB	European Federation of Societies for Ultrasound in Medicine and Biology
WFUMB	World Federation for Ultrasound in Medicine and Biology
AR	area ratio
ARFI	acoustic radiation force impulse
SE	strain elastography
SWE	shear-wave elastography
CEUS	contrast-enhanced ultrasound
AUS	atypia of undetermined significance
FLUS	follicular lesion of undetermined significance
ROI	region of interest
EI/B ratio	elastography imaging to B-mode size ratio

Author details

Andreea Borlea[1], Laura Cotoi[1], Ioana Mozos[2] and Dana Stoian[1]*

1 Department of Endocrinology, "Victor Babes University for Medicine", Timisoara, Romania

2 Department of Functional Science, "Victor Babes University for Medicine", Timisoara, Romania

*Address all correspondence to: stoian.dana@umft.ro

IntechOpen

© 2019 The Author(s). Licensee IntechOpen. This chapter is distributed under the terms of the Creative Commons Attribution License (http://creativecommons.org/licenses/by/3.0), which permits unrestricted use, distribution, and reproduction in any medium, provided the original work is properly cited.

References

[1] Lim H, Devesa SS, Sosa JA, Check D, Kitahara CM. Trends in thyroid cancer incidence and mortality in the United States, 1974-2013. Journal of the American Medical Association. 2017;**317**(13):1338-1348

[2] Andrioli M, Carzaniga C, Persani L. Standardized ultrasound report for thyroid nodules: The endocrinologist's viewpoint. European Thyroid Journal. 2013;**2**(1):37-48

[3] Pellegriti G, Frasca F, Regalbuto C, Squatrito S, Vigneri R. Worldwide increasing incidence of thyroid cancer: Update on epidemiology and risk factors. Journal of Cancer Epidemiology. 2013;**2013**:965212

[4] Gharib H, Papini E, Garber JR, Duick DS, Harrell RM, Hegedüs L, et al. American Association of clinical endocrinologists, American college of endocrinology, and Associazione Medici Endocrinologi medical guidelines for clinical practice for the diagnosis and management of thyroid nodules – 2016 update. Endocrine Practice. 2016;**22**(Suppl 1):1-60. DOI: 10.4158/EP161208.GL

[5] Popoveniuc G, Jonklaas J. Thyroid nodules. The Medical Clinics of North America. 2012;**96**(2):329-349

[6] Gregory A, Bayat M, Kumar V, Denis M, Kim BH, Webb J, et al. Differentiation of benign and malignant thyroid nodules by using comb-push ultrasound shear elastography: A preliminary two-plane view study. Academic Radiology. 2018;**25**(11):1388-1397

[7] Gharib H, Papini E, Garber JR, Duick DS, Harrell RM, Hegedüs L, et al. American Association Of Clinical Endocrinologists, American College Of Endocrinology, And Associazione Medici Endocrinologi Medical Guidelines For Clinical Practice For The Diagnosis And Management Of Thyroid Nodules – 2016 Update. Endocrine Practice. 2016;**22**(Supplement 1):1-60

[8] Remonti LR, Kramer CK, Leitão CB, Pinto LCF, Gross JL. Thyroid Ultrasound Features and Risk of Carcinoma: A Systematic Review and Meta-Analysis of Observational Studies. Thyroid. 2015;**25**(5):538-550

[9] Russ G. Risk stratification of thyroid nodules on ultrasonography with the French TI-RADS: Description and reflections. Ultrasound (Seoul, Korea). 2016;**35**(1):25-38

[10] Russ G, Bonnema SJ, Erdogan MF, Durante C, Ngu R, Leenhardt L. European thyroid association guidelines for ultrasound malignancy risk stratification of thyroid nodules in adults: The EU-TIRADS. European Thyroid Journal. 2017;**6**(5):225-237

[11] Ha EJ, Baek JH, Na DG. Risk stratification of thyroid nodules on ultrasonography: Current status and perspectives. Thyroid. 2017;**27**(12):1463-1468. DOI: 10.1089/thy.2016.0654

[12] Albair Ashamallah G, EL-Adalany MA. Risk for malignancy of thyroid nodules: Comparative study between TIRADS and US based classification system. Egyptian Journal of Radiology and Nuclear Medicine. 2016

[13] Park J-Y, Lee HJ, Jang HW, Kim HK, Yi JH, Lee W, et al. A proposal for a thyroid imaging reporting and data system for ultrasound features of thyroid carcinoma. Thyroid. 2009;**19**(11):1257-1264

[14] Kwak JY, Han KH, Yoon JH, Moon HJ, Son EJ, Park SH, et al. Thyroid

imaging reporting and data system for US features of nodules: A step in establishing better stratification of cancer risk. Radiology. 2011;**260**(3): 892-899. DOI: 10.1148/radiol.11110206

[15] Yoon JH, Lee HS, Kim E-K, Moon HJ, Kwak JY. Malignancy risk stratification of thyroid nodules: Comparison between the thyroid imaging reporting and data system and the 2014 American Thyroid Association management guidelines. Radiology. 2015;**278**(3):917-924. DOI: 10.1148/radiol.2015150056

[16] Russ G, Royer B, Bigorgne C, Rouxel A, Bienvenu-Perrard M, Leenhardt L. Prospective evaluation of thyroid imaging reporting and data system on 4550 nodules with and without elastography. European Journal of Endocrinology. 2013;**168**(5):649-655

[17] Stoian D, Timar B, Derban M, Pantea S, Varcus F, Craina M, et al. Thyroid imaging reporting and data system (TI-RADS): The impact of quantitative strain elastography for better stratification of cancer risks. Medical Ultrasonography. 2015

[18] Hoang JK, Middleton WD, Farjat AE, Langer JE, Reading CC, Teefey SA, et al. Reduction in thyroid nodule biopsies and improved accuracy with American College of Radiology Thyroid Imaging Reporting and Data System. Radiology. 2018;**287**(1):185-193. DOI: 10.1148/radiol.2018172572

[19] Haugen BR, Alexander EK, Bible KC, Doherty GM, Mandel SJ, Nikiforov YE, et al. 2015 American thyroid association management guidelines for adult patients with thyroid nodules and differentiated thyroid cancer: The American Thyroid Association guidelines task force on thyroid nodules and differentiated thyroid cancer. Thyroid. 2016;**26**(1):1-133. Available from: https://www.ncbi.nlm.nih.gov/pubmed/26462967

[20] Dean DS, Gharib H. Fine-Needle Aspiration Biopsy of the Thyroid Gland. In: De Groot LJ, Chrousos G, Dungan K, et al., editors. Endotext [Internet]. South Dartmouth (MA): MDText.com, Inc.; 2000. Available from: https://www.ncbi.nlm.nih.gov/books/NBK285544/ [Updated 2015 Apr 26]

[21] Cappelli C, Pirola I, Agosti B, Tironi A, Gandossi E, Incardona P, et al. Complications after fine-needle aspiration cytology: A retrospective study of 7449 consecutive thyroid nodules. The British Journal of Oral & Maxillofacial Surgery. 2017 Apr;**55**(3):266-269

[22] Cibas ES, Ali SZ. The 2017 Bethesda System for Reporting Thyroid Cytopathology. Journal of the American Society of Cytopathology. 2017;**6**(6):217-222

[23] Liu X, Medici M, Kwong N, Angell TE, Marqusee E, Kim MI, et al. Bethesda Categorization of Thyroid Nodule Cytology and Prediction of Thyroid Cancer Type and Prognosis. Thyroid. 2016;**26**(2):256-261

[24] Baloch ZW, Cibas ES, Clark DP, et al. The National Cancer Institute Thyroid fine needle aspiration state of the science conference: A summation. Cytojournal. 2008;**5**:6

[25] Yi KH. The Revised 2016 Korean Thyroid Association Guidelines for Thyroid Nodules and Cancers: Differences from the 2015 American Thyroid Association Guidelines. Endocrinology and Metabolism. 2016;**31**(3):373

[26] Lubitz CC, Nagarkatti SS, Faquin WC, Samir AE, Hassan MC, Barbesino G, et al. Diagnostic yield of nondiagnostic thyroid nodules is not altered by timing of repeat biopsy. Thyroid. 2012;**22**(6):590-594. Available from: https://www.ncbi.nlm.nih.gov/pubmed/22667452

[27] Sigrist RMS, Liau J, Kaffas AE, Chammas MC, Willmann JK. Ultrasound elastography: Review of techniques and clinical applications. Theranostics. 2017;7(5):1303-1329

[28] Monpeyssen H, Tramalloni J, Poirée S, Hélénon O, Correas JM. Elastography of the thyroid. Diagnostic and Interventional Imaging. 2013

[29] Dighe MK. Elastography of thyroid masses. Ultrasound Clinics. 2014;**9**(1):13-24

[30] Bamber J, Cosgrove D, Dietrich CF, Fromageau J, Bojunga J, Calliada F, et al. EFSUMB guidelines and recommendations on the clinical use of ultrasound elastography. Part 1: Basic principles and technology. Ultraschall in der Medizin. 2013;**34**(2):169-184

[31] Dietrich CF, Barr RG, Farrokh A, Dighe M, Hocke M, Jenssen C, et al. Strain elastography–How to do it? Ultrasound International Open. 2017;**3**(4):E137-E149

[32] Cosgrove D, Barr R, Bojunga J, Cantisani V, Chammas MC, Dighe M, et al. WFUMB guidelines and recommendations on the clinical use of ultrasound Elastography: Part 4. Thyroid. Ultrasound in Medicine & Biology. 2017;**43**(1):4-26

[33] Shiina T. JSUM ultrasound elastography practice guidelines: Basics and terminology. Journal of Medical Ultrasonics (2001). 2013;**40**(4):309-323

[34] Carlsen JF, Ewertsen C, Lönn L, Nielsen MB. Strain Elastography ultrasound: An overview with emphasis on breast Cancer diagnosis. Diagnostics (Basel, Switzerland). 2013;**3**(1):117-125. Available from: https://www.ncbi.nlm.nih.gov/pubmed/26835671

[35] Kwak JY, Kim E-K. Ultrasound elastography for thyroid nodules: Recent advances. Ultrasonography. 2014;**33**(2):75-82. DOI: 10.14366/usg.13025

[36] Aydin R, Elmali M, Polat AV, Danaci M, Akpolat I. Comparison of muscle-to-nodule and parenchyma-to-nodule strain ratios in the differentiation of benign and malignant thyroid nodules: Which one should we use? European Journal of Radiology. 2014;**83**(3):e131-e136

[37] Dudea SM, Botar-Jid C. Ultrasound elastography in thyroid disease. Medical Ultrasonography. 2015;**17**(1):74-96

[38] Cantisani V, D'Andrea V, Biancari F, Medvedyeva O, Di Segni M, Olive M, et al. Prospective evaluation of multiparametric ultrasound and quantitative elastosonography in the differential diagnosis of benign and malignant thyroid nodules: Preliminary experience. European Journal of Radiology. 2012;**81**(10):2678-2683

[39] Cantisani V, Maceroni P, D'Andrea V, Patrizi G, Di Segni M, De Vito C, et al. Strain ratio ultrasound elastography increases the accuracy of colour-Doppler ultrasound in the evaluation of Thy-3 nodules. A bi-Centre university experience. European Radiology. 2016;**26**(5):1441-1449

[40] Ding J, Cheng H, Ning C, Huang J, Zhang Y. Quantitative measurement for thyroid cancer characterization based on elastography. Journal of Ultrasound in Medicine. 2011;**30**(9):1259-1266. DOI: 10.7863/jum.2011.30.9.1259

[41] Xing P, Wu L, Zhang C, Li S, Liu C, Wu C. Differentiation of benign from malignant thyroid lesions. Journal of Ultrasound in Medicine. 2011;**30**(5):663-669. DOI: 10.7863/jum.2011.30.5.663

[42] Barr RG. Real-time ultrasound elasticity of the breast: Initial clinical results. Ultrasound Quarterly. 2010;**26**(2):61-66

[43] Zhang F-J, Han R-L, Zhao X-M. The value of virtual touch tissue image (VTI) and virtual touch tissue quantification (VTQ) in the differential diagnosis of thyroid nodules. European Journal of Radiology. 2014;**83**(11):2033-2040. DOI: 10.1016/j.ejrad.2014.08.011

[44] Lim D-J, Luo S, Kim M-H, Ko S-H, Kim Y. Interobserver agreement and intraobserver reproducibility in thyroid ultrasound elastography. American Journal of Roentgenology. 2012;**198**(4):896-901. DOI: 10.2214/AJR.11.7009

[45] Bojunga J, Herrmann E, Meyer G, Weber S, Zeuzem S, Friedrich-Rust M. Real-time elastography for the differentiation of benign and malignant thyroid nodules: A meta-analysis. Thyroid. 2010;**20**(10):1145-1150

[46] Rago T, Scutari M, Santini F, Loiacono V, Piaggi P, Di Coscio G, et al. Real-time elastosonography: Useful tool for refining the presurgical diagnosis in thyroid nodules with indeterminate or nondiagnostic cytology. The Journal of Clinical Endocrinology and Metabolism. 2010;**95**(12):5274-5280. DOI: 10.1210/jc.2010-0901

[47] Trimboli P, Guglielmi R, Monti S, Misischi I, Graziano F, Nasrollah N, et al. Ultrasound sensitivity for thyroid malignancy is increased by real-time elastography: A prospective multicenter study. The Journal of Clinical Endocrinology and Metabolism. 2012;**97**(12):4524-4530

[48] Nell S, Kist JW, Debray TPA, de Keizer B, van Oostenbrugge TJ, Borel Rinkes IHM, et al. Qualitative elastography can replace thyroid nodule fine-needle aspiration in patients with soft thyroid nodules. A systematic review and meta-analysis. European Journal of Radiology. 2015;**84**(4):652-661

[49] Hu X, Liu Y, Qian L. Diagnostic potential of real-time elastography (RTE) and shear wave elastography (SWE) to differentiate benign and malignant thyroid nodules: A systematic review and meta-analysis. Medicine (Baltimore). 2017;**96**(43):e8282-e8282. Available from: https://www.ncbi.nlm.nih.gov/pubmed/29068996

[50] Hong Y, Wu Y, Luo Z, Wu N, Liu X. Impact of nodular size on the predictive values of gray-scale, color-Doppler ultrasound, and sonoelastography for assessment of thyroid nodules. Journal of Zhejiang University. Science. B. 2012;**13**(9):707-716. Available from: https://www.ncbi.nlm.nih.gov/pubmed/22949361

[51] Oliver C, Vaillant-Lombard J, Albarel F, Berbis J, Veyrieres JB, Sebag F, et al. What is the contribution of elastography to thyroid nodules evaluation? Annales d'Endocrinologie. 2011;**72**(2):120-124

[52] Tatar IG, Kurt A, Yilmaz KB, Akinci M, Kulacoglu H, Hekimoglu B. The learning curve of real time elastosonography: A preliminary study conducted for the assessment of malignancy risk in thyroid nodules. Medical Ultrasonography. 2013;**15**(4):278-284

[53] Cantisani V, Grazhdani H, Drakonaki E, D'Andrea V, Segni MD, Kaleshi E, et al. Strain US Elastography for the Characterization of Thyroid Nodules: Advantages and Limitation. International Journal of Endocrinology. 2015;**2015**:1-8

[54] Nowicki A, Dobruch-Sobczak K. Introduction to ultrasound elastography. Journal of Ultrasonography. 2016;**16**(65):113-124

[55] Zhan J, Jin J-M, Diao X-H, Chen Y. Acoustic radiation force impulse imaging (ARFI) for differentiation of benign and malignant thyroid nodules–A

meta-analysis. European Journal of Radiology. 2015;**84**(11):2181-2186. DOI: 10.1016/j.ejrad.2015.07.015

[56] Dong F-J, Li M, Jiao Y, Xu J-F, Xiong Y, Zhang L, et al. Acoustic radiation force impulse imaging for detecting thyroid nodules: A systematic review and pooled meta-analysis. Medical Ultrasonography. 2015;**17**(2):192-199

[57] Lin P, Chen M, Liu B, Wang S, Li X. Diagnostic performance of shear wave elastography in the identification of malignant thyroid nodules: A meta-analysis. European Radiology. 2014;**24**(11):2729-2738

[58] Park AY, Son EJ, Han K, Youk JH, Kim J-A, Park CS. Shear wave elastography of thyroid nodules for the prediction of malignancy in a large scale study. European Journal of Radiology. 2015;**84**(3):407-412. DOI: 10.1016/j.ejrad.2014.11.019

[59] Zhang Y-F, Xu H-X, He Y, Liu C, Guo L-H, Liu L-N, et al. Virtual touch tissue quantification of acoustic radiation force impulse: A new ultrasound elastic imaging in the diagnosis of thyroid nodules. PLoS One. 2012;**7**(11):e49094

[60] Hou X-J, Sun A-X, Zhou X-L, Ji Q, Wang H-B, Wei H, et al. The application of virtual touch tissue quantification (VTQ) in diagnosis of thyroid lesions: A preliminary study. European Journal of Radiology. 2013;**82**(5):797-801

[61] Han R, Li F, Wang Y, Ying Z, Zhang Y. Virtual touch tissue quantification (VTQ) in the diagnosis of thyroid nodules with coexistent chronic autoimmune Hashimoto's thyroiditis: A preliminary study. European Journal of Radiology. 2015;**84**(2):327-331

[62] Friedrich-Rust M, Romenski O, Meyer G, Dauth N, Holzer K, Grunwald F, et al. Acoustic radiation force impulse-imaging for the evaluation of the thyroid gland: A limited patient feasibility study. Ultrasonics. 2012;**52**(1):69-74

[63] Bojunga J, Dauth N, Berner C, Meyer G, Holzer K, Voelkl L, et al. Acoustic radiation force impulse imaging for differentiation of thyroid nodules. PLoS One. 2012;**7**(8):e42735

[64] Grazhdani H, Cantisani V, Lodise P, Di Rocco G, Proietto MC, Fioravanti E, et al. Prospective evaluation of acoustic radiation force impulse technology in the differentiation of thyroid nodules: Accuracy and interobserver variability assessment. Journal of Ultrasound. 2014;**17**(1):13-20

[65] Samir AE, Dhyani M, Anvari A, Prescott J, Halpern EF, Faquin WC, et al. Shear-wave elastography for the preoperative risk stratification of follicular-patterned lesions of the thyroid: Diagnostic accuracy and optimal measurement plane. Radiology. 2015;**277**(2):565-573

[66] Tian W, Hao S, Gao B, Jiang Y, Zhang X, Zhang S, et al. Comparing the diagnostic accuracy of RTE and SWE in differentiating malignant thyroid nodules from benign ones: A meta-analysis. Cellular Physiology and Biochemistry. 2016;**39**(6):2451-2463

[67] Liu B-X, Xie X-Y, Liang J-Y, Zheng Y-L, Huang G-L, Zhou L-Y, et al. Shear wave elastography versus real-time elastography on evaluation thyroid nodules: A preliminary study. European Journal of Radiology. 2014;**83**(7):1135-1143. DOI: 10.1016/j.ejrad.2014.02.024

[68] Gay S, Schiaffino S, Santamorena G, Massa B, Ansaldo G, Turtulici G, et al. Role of strain elastography and shear-wave elastography in a multiparametric clinical approach to indeterminate cytology thyroid nodules. Medical Science Monitor. 2018;**24**:6273-6279. Available from: https://www.ncbi.nlm.nih.gov/pubmed/30194820

[69] Kuru B, Atmaca A, Kefeli M. Malignancy rate associated with Bethesda category III (AUS/FLUS) with and without repeat fine needle aspiration biopsy. Diagnostic Cytopathology. 2016;**44**(5):394-398

[70] Sahli ZT, Smith PW, Umbricht CB, Zeiger MA. Preoperative molecular markers in thyroid nodules. Frontiers in Endocrinology (Lausanne). 2018;**9**:179

[71] Ward LS, Kloos RT. Molecular markers in the diagnosis of thyroid nodules. Arquivos Brasileiros de Endocrinologia e Metabologia. 2013;**57**(2):89-97

[72] Zhang M, Lin O. Molecular testing of thyroid nodules: A review of current available tests for fine-needle aspiration specimens. Archives of Pathology & Laboratory Medicine. 2016;**140**(12):1338-1344. DOI: 10.5858/arpa.2016-0100-RA

[73] Alexander EK, Kennedy GC, Baloch ZW, Cibas ES, Chudova D, Diggans J, et al. Preoperative diagnosis of benign thyroid nodules with indeterminate cytology. The New England Journal of Medicine. 2012;**367**(8):705-715

[74] Labourier E, Shifrin A, Busseniers AE, Lupo MA, Manganelli ML, Andruss B, et al. Molecular testing for miRNA, mRNA, and DNA on fine-needle aspiration improves the preoperative diagnosis of thyroid nodules with indeterminate cytology. The Journal of Clinical Endocrinology and Metabolism. 2015;**100**(7):2743-2750

[75] Nikiforov YE, Carty SE, Chiosea SI, Coyne C, Duvvuri U, Ferris RL, et al. Highly accurate diagnosis of cancer in thyroid nodules with follicular neoplasm/suspicious for a follicular neoplasm cytology by ThyroSeq v2 next-generation sequencing assay. Cancer. 2014;**120**(23):3627-3634

[76] Liu R, Hao S, Zhang H, Ma J, Liu X, Xu J, et al. Correlation of thyroid stimulating hormone receptor mRNA expression levels in peripheral blood with undesirable clinicopathological features in papillary thyroid carcinoma patients. Oncotarget. 2017;**8**(43):74129-74138. Available from: https://www.ncbi.nlm.nih.gov/pubmed/29088773

[77] Wagner K, Arciaga R, Siperstein A, Milas M, Warshawsky I, Sethu S, et al. Thyrotropin receptor/thyroglobulin messenger ribonucleic acid in peripheral blood and fine-needle aspiration cytology: Diagnostic synergy for detecting thyroid cancer. The Journal of Clinical Endocrinology and Metabolism. 2005;**90**(4):1921-1924. DOI: 10.1210/jc.2004-1793

[78] Lippolis PV, Tognini S, Materazzi G, Polini A, Mancini R, Ambrosini CE, et al. Is elastography actually useful in the presurgical selection of thyroid nodules with indeterminate cytology? The Journal of Clinical Endocrinology and Metabolism. 2011;**96**(11):E1826-E1830. DOI: 10.1210/jc.2011-1021

[79] Azizi G, Keller JM, Mayo ML, Piper K, Puett D, Earp KM, et al. Shear wave elastography and AfirmaTM gene expression classifier in thyroid nodules with indeterminate cytology: A comparison study. Endocrine. 2018;**59**(3):573-584. Available from: https://www.ncbi.nlm.nih.gov/pubmed/29350311

[80] Zhan J, Ding H. Application of contrast-enhanced ultrasound for evaluation of thyroid nodules. Ultrasound (Seoul, Korea). 2018;**37**(4):288-297. Available from: https://www.ncbi.nlm.nih.gov/pubmed/30213158

[81] Nolsøe CP, Lorentzen T. International guidelines for contrast-enhanced ultrasonography: Ultrasound imaging in the new millennium. Ultrasound (Seoul, Korea). 2016;**35**(2):89-103. Available

from: https://www.ncbi.nlm.nih.gov/pubmed/26867761

[82] Galiè M, D'Onofrio M, Montani M, Amici A, Calderan L, Marzola P, et al. Tumor vessel compression hinders perfusion of ultrasonographic contrast agents. Neoplasia. 2005;**7**(5):528-536. Available from: https://www.ncbi.nlm.nih.gov/pubmed/15967105

[83] Cantisani V, Consorti F, Guerrisi A, Guerrisi I, Ricci P, Di Segni M, et al. Prospective comparative evaluation of quantitative-elastosonography (Q-elastography) and contrast-enhanced ultrasound for the evaluation of thyroid nodules: Preliminary experience. European Journal of Radiology. 2013;**82**(11):1892-1898

[84] Jiang J, Shang X, Wang H, Xu Y-B, Gao Y, Zhou Q. Diagnostic value of contrast-enhanced ultrasound in thyroid nodules with calcification. The Kaohsiung Journal of Medical Sciences. 2015;**31**(3):138-144

[85] Wu Q, Wang Y, Li Y, Hu B, He Z-Y. Diagnostic value of contrast-enhanced ultrasound in solid thyroid nodules with and without enhancement. Endocrine. 2016;**53**(2):480-488

[86] Wiesinger I, Kroiss E, Zausig N, Hornung M, Zeman F, Stroszczynski C, et al. Analysis of arterial dynamic micro-vascularization with contrast-enhanced ultrasound (CEUS) in thyroid lesions using external perfusion software: First results. Clinical Hemorheology and Microcirculation. 2016;**64**(4):747-755

[87] Sun B, Lang L, Zhu X, Jiang F, Hong Y, He L. Accuracy of contrast-enhanced ultrasound in the identification of thyroid nodules: A meta-analysis. International Journal of Clinical and Experimental Medicine. 2015;**8**(8):12882-12889

[88] Yu D, Han Y, Chen T. Contrast-enhanced ultrasound for differentiation of benign and malignant thyroid lesions: Meta-analysis. Otolaryngology and Head and Neck Surgery. 2014;**151**(6):909-915

[89] Zhan J, Diao X-H, Chen L, Jin J-M, Chen Y. Role of contrast-enhanced ultrasound in diagnosis of thyroid nodules in acoustic radiation force impulse "Gray Zone". Ultrasound in Medicine & Biology. 2017;**43**(6):1179-1186. DOI: 10.1016/j.ultrasmedbio.2017.02.006

[90] Menzilcioglu MS, Duymus M, Avcu S. Sonographic elastography of the thyroid gland. Polish Journal of Radiology. 2016;**81**:152-156. Available from: https://www.ncbi.nlm.nih.gov/pubmed/27103947

[91] Mehrotra P, McQueen A, Kolla S, Johnson SJ, Richardson DL. Does elastography reduce the need for thyroid FNAs? Clinical Endocrinology. 2012;**78**(6):942-949. DOI: 10.1111/cen.12077

Chapter 4

Papillary Thyroid Carcinoma Intertwined with Hashimoto's Thyroiditis: An Intriguing Correlation

Maria V. Deligiorgi and Dimitrios T. Trafalis

Abstract

Illustrating the ancient link connecting inflammation with cancer, the correlation of papillary thyroid carcinoma (PTC) with Hashimoto's thyroiditis (HT) has long been pursued as intersection of autoimmunity-induced chronic inflammation and tumor-induced immunity. The dramatic rise of the incidence of PTC over the last decades—the main culprit for "thyroid cancer (TC) epidemic"—parallels the increasing incidence of HT, potentially reflecting a pathogenetic link that could be harnessed in diagnostics and therapeutics. Prompted by this perspective, in the present chapter, we dissect the hitherto elusive interrelationship of PTC with HT, focusing on four issues: firstly, an unresolved conundrum is whether PTC emerges due to or notwithstanding immune response or mirrors the "tumor defense-induced autoimmunity." Secondly, the interrelationship of HT with PTC may be merely epiphenomenon of selection bias inherent in thyroidectomy series. Thirdly, the impact of HT on coexistent PTC is equivocal—host protective versus tumor protective. Fourthly, translating serum concentrations of thyroid autoantibodies and thyroid-stimulating hormone (TSH) into predictive and prognostic PTC biomarkers dichotomizes, till now, the researchers. In the era of precision medicine, illuminating whether HT precipitates PTC or *vice versa* is awaited with anticipation in order to refine the preventive and therapeutic policy counteracting "TC epidemic."

Keywords: papillary thyroid carcinoma, hashimoto's thyroiditis, anti-thyroglobulin autoantibodies, anti-thyroperoxidase autoantibodies, thyroid-stimulating hormone

1. Introduction

Initially reported by Dailey et al. in 1955, the correlation of papillary thyroid carcinoma (PTC)—the most common thyroid cancer (TC) histotype—with Hashimoto's thyroiditis (HT) [1] has long been pursued, rekindling the ancient link between inflammation and cancer [2]. Bearing in mind the rising incidence of PTC over the last decades [3], establishing causality between PTC and HT—an issue highly contested—could lay the groundwork for a preventive policy. Moreover, harnessing the interrelationship of PTC with HT could refine therapeutics with respect to PTC. The present chapter dissects the correlation of PTC with HT, delving into a strongly insinuated immunological link. A comprehensive review of current literature emphasizes on the bewildering clinical significance of the interrelationship of PTC with HT. The intriguing predictive and prognostic value of serum concentrations of thyroid autoantibodies and thyroid-stimulating hormone (TSH) in the context of PTC coexistent with HT paints a more nuanced and sophisticated picture.

2. Tailoring the treatment of PTC: where does coexistent HT stand?

Thyroid cancer (TC) is the most common endocrine malignancy [4], though comprising only 2.1% of global cancer burden [5]. It is estimated that 52,070 new TC cases will occur in 2019 in the United States, while 2170 patients will die of this cancer type [6]. Derived from follicular epithelial cells, PTC constitutes the most common TC subtype in iodine sufficient areas, accounting for 85% of differentiated TC (DTC) [7] and 70–80% of TC [8]. In light of the interface between "TC epidemic" and "epidemic of diagnosis," a true increase of the incidence of PTC due to environmental, hormonal, and lifestyle risk factors appears to be merged with overdiagnosis of subclinical disease owing to meticulous screening [3, 9–11].

The indolent nature of PTC imposes a paradigm shift from ameliorating 10-year survival rates exceeding 90% to eliminating the recurrence incidence that hovers at 15–30% [12]. Individualization of therapeutic approach is deemed to confront the emerging challenges [13]. Seminal studies [4, 14, 15] recently illuminated the "dark matter" of the previously unidentified driver genetic events in 96% of PTC [4], being translated into molecular-based risk-adapted therapeutic strategies [7]. Although surgery is the cornerstone of treatment of PTC, a tailored approach with respect to the extent of thyroidectomy and lymph node dissection, the radioiodine ablation, and the management of radioiodine-refractory recurrent/metastatic disease has been endorsed [7].

Provided that the clinical relevance of the increasingly reported interrelationship of PTC with HT is clarified, the incorporation thereof in current PTC risk stratification systems may empower a personalized treatment. This perspective is anticipated to build on accomplishing a fine-tuned balance in terms of decision-making concerning PTC, precluding both overestimating an innocent disease and ignoring a metastatic potential.

3. HT at a glance

HT, originally designated as "struma lymphomatosa" by Dr. Hakaru Hashimoto in 1912 [16], is the most common autoimmune thyroid disease and the most common cause of hypothyroidism in iodine sufficient areas, showing a worldwide annual incidence varying from 0.3 to 1.5 cases per 1000 individuals [17]. An insightful approach concerning the multifactorial etiology of HT has been proposed by Weetman et al.: aligned in a way reminiscent of the wholes of the Swiss cheese are genetic factors acting as susceptibility loci—major histocompatibility human leukocyte antigen (HLA) genes, immunoregulatory genes, thyroid specific genes-environmental factors—excess iodine intake, viral infections, stress, endocrine disruptors—as well as non-modifiable intrinsic factors—female sex, parity, age. Traversed by a hypothetical arrow, this conceivable line translates in a catastrophic event [18].

The histopathologically confirmed HT is characterized by diffuse lymphocytic infiltrate, formation of lymphoid follicles with germinal centers within normal thyroid tissue [19], and, potentially, atrophy of parenchymal tissue gradually replaced by fibrous tissue [20]. The identification of the autoantibodies hallmark of HT in 1936 [21] paved the way for Rose and Witebsky to designate HT as the archetype of autoimmune destructive disorders [22]. Whereas the pathogenesis of HT is unclear, crucial is considered the imbalance between T-helper (Th)2 cells—Th CD (cluster of differentiation)4+ cells credited with stimulation of B cells, which in turn produce thyroid autoantibodies- and Th1 cells-cytotoxic Th CD4+ cells directly attacking the thyroid follicular cells. This concept has been refined by the imbalance between Th17 cells and Th cells producing mainly IL-17, involved also in carcinomas- and T regulatory (Treg) cells-Th CD4+ cells deemed to halt the immune response [23]. Especially, an increased TH17/Treg ratio ascribed to both enhancement of TH17 expression and decrease of Treg is involved in the pathogenesis of HT [24]. Incriminated for the depletion of thyrocytes in HT is principally the autocrine/paracrine Fas-/Fas ligand (FasL)-induced extrinsic apoptotic pathway [24, 25].

4. Rationality in the investigation of the interrelationship of PTC with HT

Apart from the well-established connection of HT with thyroid lymphoma [26], which is beyond the scope of the present chapter, the association of TC with HT concerns almost exclusively the PTC [27], alluding to a discriminating, though unknown, pathogenetic link.

Since PTC is conceived as the main culprit for the explosive rise of TC incidence [3], the hypothesis that the increasing incidence of HT hastens the "TC epidemic" is appealing. Considering that the inflammation has been envisaged as the "seventh hallmark of cancer" [28], the autoimmunity-induced inflammatory milieu [29] merits further interrogation as the missing piece in the puzzle of the interrelationship of PTC with HT.

An alternative explanation that cannot be ruled out is that third extraneous variables actually cause the coexistence of PTC with HT. Indeed, both PTC and HT are precipitated by an interplay among genetic factors and environmental influences most of which are shared by the two entities. Emphasis is placed on risk factors implicated in the pathogenesis of both PTC and HT, such as female predominance, excess iodine intake, and exposure to radiation [30–34], implying a spurious correlation.

Nonetheless, a common origin of PTC and HT from cancer stem cells expressing p63 proteins—homologs of p53 proteins postulated to regulate squamous stem cell commitment—has been suggested. In fact, the cancer stem cells constitute pluripotent cells deemed to remain undifferentiated or undergo benign squamoid and glandural maturation or be differentiated to follicular epithelial cells, harboring the potential to elicit both PTC and HT [35, 36].

The interrelationship of PTC with HT spurs a realm of intense research, principally in four respects. Firstly, the pathogenetic link between HT and PTC remains elusive; however, accumulative evidence suggests that these two entities are immunologically linked [29]. Secondly, some authors argue that this interrelationship is merely epiphenomenon of selection bias inherent in studies encompassing surgical series [37, 38]. Thirdly, equivocal—favorable versus unfavorable—is the impact of HT on the prognosis of concurrent PTC [39–48]. Finally, the translation of the serum concentrations of thyroid autoantibodies [49–56] and thyroid-stimulating hormone (TSH) [55, 57–63] into predictive and prognostic PTC biomarkers incites a perpetual conflict.

5. Exploring the immunological link between PTC and HT

Compelling evidence insinuate that the PTC and the HT represent two extremes in the continuum of immune response. In cancer, dominant is an anti-inflammatory response dictated by cancer cells per se, counteracting the antitumor immune surveillance. Quite the contrary, an overactivated inflammatory response owing to breakage of self-tolerance attacks host tissue cells, resulting in tissue damage in the context of autoimmune diseases. Despite the fundamental differences between the tumor microenvironment and the autoimmune milieu, certain parallel aspects of these two landscapes have been recognized [64]. For instance, the macrophages (M) and the neutrophils (N)—cells of myeloid origin—are encountered in both cancer and autoimmunity that act as well-coordinated partners to orchestrate the innate immune attack. Showing plasticity, these cells transition from proinflammatory M1/N1 polarization, devoted to kill pathogens or cancer cells, to anti-inflammatory M2/N2 polarization, dedicated to repair tissue damage and promote angiogenesis. A shift toward M2 macrophage polarization is a core component of tumor microenvironment, observed in autoimmune milieu as well, providing a hint to the interface thereof. Furthermore, supportive of the tumor-promoting M2 macrophage polarization is the local hypoxic milieu inherent in both autoimmune and cancerous diseases [64].

The elucidation of the continuum of immune response could provide insights into the pathogenetic background of the coexistence of PTC with HT. Given that the macrophage phenotype M2 is considered tumor-promoting contrary to the antitumor effect of M1 phenotype, an appealing hypothesis connecting PTC with HT is derived from the intrathyroidal immune profiling of euthyroid HT conducted very recently by Imam et al. [65]. The immune infiltrate in euthyroid HT proved to contain low count of natural killer (NK) cells, facilitating the differentiation of the macrophage phenotype M0 to the M2 phenotype, which in concert with the observed low count of M1 macrophages may interpret the higher risk of PTC inherent in euthyroid HT [65].

Interestingly, overexpression of Toll-like receptors (TLR)—cell surface receptors credited with recognition of pathogen-related molecules, crucial for activation of innate and adaptive immunity—is detected immunohistochemically in human thyrocytes surrounded by immune cells in all patients with HT. The high basal TLR3 mRNA levels observed in PTC, reinforcing the shared immunological landscape, are consistent [66, 67].

Dissecting the interface of HT with PTC is expected to unveil novel targets for immunomodulation. For instance, triggering the innate immunity via the TLR5 agonist flagellin, being already in clinical trials as inducer of NK activation [68], could be interrogated as a modality to reverse the M2 macrophage phenotype in PTC coexistent with HT.

In pursuit of the immunological link connecting PTC with HT, three hypotheses, rather interrelated, shape a conceptual framework outlined below.

5.1 Thyroid malignancy develops despite immune response in the context of HT

Manifold mechanisms have been proposed to underlie the escape of PTC cells from immune response in the context of autoimmunity: (i) the ability of PTC cells to manipulate the expression of immune-regulatory cytokines, editing the immune response; (ii) the enhancement of Treg known to suppress the NK cell effector functions, mainly the cytotoxicity; and (iii) the promotion of expression of specific surface molecules facilitating tumor development and growth, such as the membrane-bound transforming growth factor b (TGFb), histocompatibility antigen, class 1, G (HLA-G), FasL, and B7 homolog 1(B7H1) [28].

Moreover, the interrelationship of PTC with HT may empower the escape of cancer cells from immune surveillance, consolidating the dogma that "cancer is a wound that never heals since tumor cells hijack the wound healing machinery for their own gain" [69]. In fact, a recently discovered "unexpected player", the T cell double negative (DN) CD4(−) CD8(−), expressed both in PTC and in thyroid autoimmunity, downregulates the proliferation of activated T effector cells and the cytokine production, fostering an immunosuppressive microenvironment [70]. Favoring immune tolerance, the FOXP3+ Treg cells—crucial players of thyroid autoimmunity [71]—are encountered also in PTC [70]. The dendritic cells (DCs), beyond governing the autoimmune milieu, are also expressed in PTC, being responsible for the expansion of FOXP3+ Treg cells, allowing the tumor immune evasion and, thus, enabling the PTC progression [72].

5.2 Thyroid malignancy develops owing to thyroid autoimmunity

The first detection of lymphocytes in neoplastic tissues by Virchow in 1863 [73] paved the way for the endorsement of chronic inflammation as a precipitating factor for certain cancer types. In that respect, thyroid gland could be conceived as an intersection of HT-induced chronic inflammation and cancer; however, a causal relationship is yet to be defined. In light of the cancer-related inflammation (CRI), the concurrence of PTC with HT might reflect either the malignant transformation ascribed to an autoimmunity-induced chronic inflammatory milieu (extrinsic pathway) or the inflammatory response to tumor (intrinsic pathway) [74].

The perpetually overactive immune response in the context of HT initiates an inflammatory vicious cycle with the potential to gear the journey of normal cells toward malignancy, rendering the interrelationship of PTC with HT the epitome of the extrinsic pathway of CRI [74].

Central in the extrinsic pathway is the "smoldering inflammation," an ungoverned inflammatory milieu orchestrated by immune/inflammatory cells, involving macrophages, immature DCs, and mast cells, expressing a myriad of cytokines, chemokines, and growth factors, such as interleukin (IL)-1b, tumor necrosis factor a (TNFa), IL-6, (C-C motif) ligand 2 (CCL2)/monocyte chemoattractant protein 1 (MCP-1), CXC chemokine ligand (CXCL8)/IL-8, vascular endothelial growth factor (VEGF), as well as reactive oxygen species (ROS) and reactive nitrogen species (RNS), spurring tissue damage, neo-angiogenesis, and tissue remodeling [75, 76]. Implicated in this milieu is the hypoxic microenvironment, inherent in both PTC and HT, favoring the progression of tumor, reinforcing, among others, the neo-angiogenesis and the shift of metabolism toward anaerobic glycolysis [64].

Overexpression of cyclooxygenase-2 (COX-2)—an enzyme involved in initiation [77] and progression of thyroid tumors [78]—and inducible nitric oxide synthases (iNOS), key elements of CRI, has been observed in epithelial cells of lymphocytic thyroiditis, follicular adenoma, and PTC contrary to the absence or the limited expression thereof in normal thyroid epithelium, potentially linking carcinogenesis to autoimmunity [79].

Intertwined with the extrinsic pathway is the intrinsic pathway: genetic alterations caused by DNA damage induced by the "smoldering inflammation" [80] trigger a proinflammatory transcriptional program [74]. For instance, the oncogene RAS is involved in the induction of chemokine CXCL8 [75], an inflammatory mediator of both cancer [75] and autoimmunity [64]. Moreover, phosphatase and tensin homolog (PTEN) mutation, a key element of the oncogenic phosphoinositide 3-kinase (PI3K)/protein kinase B (AKT) pathway, leads to upregulation of hypoxia-inducible factor-1 (HIF1), which, in turn, upregulates the CXC chemokine receptor 4 (CXCR4) [75], well-recognized player of autoimmunity [81]. Accordingly, the observed activation of the PI3K/AKT pathway in HT, PTC, and HT coexistent with PTC contrary to the absence of activation thereof in normal follicles is rational [82].

Illustrating the common molecular background shared by PTC and HT, the rearranged during transfection (RET)/PTC rearrangements—landmarks of PTC—are detected in 95% of HT [83]. Moreover, the RET/PTC1 rearrangement has been detected more frequently in PTC coexistent with autoimmunity than PTC alone (31% versus 13%, respectively) [84]. The inflammatory milieu fosters the genesis of RET/PTC rearrangements either via secreting ROS and RNS [85]—the main culprit for mutagenic-mediated DNA damage [2]—or sustaining the survival of thyroid cells that harbor RET/PTC rearrangements.

The oncogenic RET/PTC-RAS-BRAF-mitogen-activated protein kinase (MAPK) cascade [74] may connect the oxyphil cell metaplasia of HT with PTC, considering the enhancement of the expression of RET, nuclear RAS, and extracellular signal-regulated kinases (ERKs)—core components of MAPK cascade—not only in PTC but also in oxyphil cells in the context of HT [86].

Further, experimental data unravel that the RET/PTC1 exogenously expressed on normal human thyroid cells induces an inflammatory milieu involving crucial chemokines and their receptors, promoting functions vital for tumor progression, such as proliferation and survival of cancer cells [e.g., CXCR4/CXCL1] as well as neo-angiogenesis (e.g., CXL1, 2, 3, 5, 6, and 8) [87].

Additionally, a constellation of RET/PTC1-induced molecules fosters the genesis and evolution of cancer, including (i) matrix metalloproteinases (MMPs) and dipeptidyl peptidase IV (DPP IV), molecules crucial for tissue remodeling, tumor invasiveness, and neo-angiogenesis [87]; (ii) urokinase-type plasminogen activator (UPA) and urokinase-type plasminogen activator receptor (UPAR), involved in cancer progression and metastasis [87]; (iii) L-selectin [87], an adhesion molecule facilitating metastasis [88]; and (iv) osteopontin (OPN) and CD44, implicated in proliferation and invasion of transformed PCCl 3 cells, rat thyroid follicular cells [89].

An intriguing RET/PTC3-induced mechanism pivotal for tumor progression is the recruitment of CD11b+Gr1+ myeloid-derived suppressor cells, providing cancer cells with the advantage of evading immune surveillance [90, 91].

However, skepticism raise the technical limitations of the applied PCR techniques and the lack of reproducibility of the results of studies detecting the RET/PTC rearrangements in HT [92]. Furthermore, the equivocal nature of RET/PTC-induced transcriptional program—tumor-promoting versus antitumor—should be considered [87].

5.3 The immune attack against PTC triggers thyroid autoimmunity

The association of PTC with HT seems more intricate than initially conceived in view of a seminal cyclic model governed by the overactive immune response, acting as a driving force for carcinogenesis, while being also a marker of tumor immunity [93]. An assumption that merits further exploration is whether the cross reaction of antitumor immunity with normal thyrocytes may precipitate HT in PTC patients genetically predisposed to thyroid autoimmunity, consolidating the hypothesis of "tumor defense-induced autoimmunity" [29]. With the advent of the era of cancer immunotherapy, new light on the coexistence of HT with PTC is shed by the increasingly reported development of HT as an adverse event of the monoclonal antibodies blocking programmed cell death (PD) protein 1 (PD-1) and PD ligand 1 (PD-L1). This revolutionary anticancer treatment unleashes the antitumor immunity at the expense of abrogating the self-tolerance, exemplifying the "tumor defense-induced" immunity [94]. For instance, a loss of circulatory PD1+ CD4+ and CD8+ T cells, an increase in peripheral CD56+CD16+ NK cells and an increase in activated monocytes have been implicated in pembrolizumab (anti-PD1 monoclonal antibody)-induced thyroiditis [94].

6. Does the coexistence of HT with PTC really exist?

An issue of major concern is whether the coexistence of PTC with HT is real or a myth nurtured by methodological pitfalls implicit in studies addressing this issue.

The great variety of the incidence of the coexistence of PTC with HT ranging from 0.5 to 38% [95] or, alternatively, from 5 to 85% is noticeable [96]. The results of the meta-analyses addressing the coexistence of PTC with HT are highly divergent [40, 48, 96, 97], as depicted in **Table 1.** The broad array of the mean rate of PTC among patients with HT extending from 1.1 to 40.1% blurs the landscape [97]. Nevertheless, according to a systematic review, the correlation of PTC with HT is statistically significant with a relative risk (RR) of HT among PTC equal to 2.36 and a RR of PTC among HT equal to 1.40 [98].

In an attempt to annotate the diverse epidemiological profile of the coexistence of PTC with HT, attention should be paid to the discrepancy among pertinent studies concerning the design, the enrolled populations, and the histopathologic definitions of HT [99]. Moreover, certain caveats hamper hitherto the interpretation of the lymphocytic infiltration and the positivity of thyroid autoantibodies. Firstly, thyroid lymphocytic infiltration confirmed on histology has been significantly associated with PTC even in the absence of thyroid autoantibodies [100]. Secondly, the pattern of Tg recognition by anti-thyroglobulin autoantibodies (TgAbs) differs between autoimmune and non-autoimmune thyroid disorders, being more restricted in autoimmune disorders as compared with nodular goiter and PTC harboring no thyroid lymphocytic infiltration [101]. However, in PTC correlated with histopathologically confirmed HT, the pattern of Tg recognition does not differ from that observed in HT [101]. Thirdly, it should be mentioned that the thyroid autoantibodies may be detected in healthy individuals [102]. Finally, the discordance among available TgAbs assays should be considered [103].

Another hurdle in evaluating the coexistence of PTC with HT is the selection bias inherent in data derived from surgical specimens wherein the prevalence of PTC is a priori higher than that in fine needle aspiration biopsy (FNAB) studies.

Reference	Results
Moon et al. [48]	PTC coexistent with HT is negatively associated with ETE (OR: 0.74, 95% CI, 0.68–0.81), LNM (OR: 0.82, 95% CI, 0.72–0.94), distant metastasis (OR: 0.49, 95% CI, 0.32–0.76), and recurrence (RR: 0.50, 95% CI, 0.41–0.61)
Lee et al. [96]	Frequency of HT in PTC: ≈23% 2.8 times higher occurrence rate of HT in PTC than in benign thyroid diseases ($p < 0.001$) 2.4 times higher incidence of HT in PTC than in other TC ($p < 0.001$) Significant association of PTC concurrent with HT with female sex (OR: 2.7; $p < 0.001$), multifocality (OR: 1.5, $p = 0.010$), absence of ETE (OR: 1.3, $p = 0.002$) and LNM (OR: 1.3, $p = 0.041$), long recurrence-free survival (HR: 0.6, $p = 0.001$)
Lai et al. [97]	Range of mean rate of PTC among patients with HT: 1.12–40.11% Overall pooled OR of PTC risk for HT (HT versus non-HT): 2.12 (95% CI, 1.78–2.52)
Singh et al. [40]	2.77 times elevated rate of PTC in patients with HT compared with control population (OR: 2.77, 95% CI, 1.24–6.21) 1.89 times higher rate of HT in patients with PTC compared with other TC types (OR: 1.89, 95% CI, 1.02–3.50) Increased PTC-free survival in patients with coexistent HT (r: 0.08, 95% CI, 0.05–0.12) Increased overall survival in PTC patients with coexistent HT (r: 0.11; 95% CI, 0.07–0.14)

Abbreviations: CI, confidence interval; ETE, extrathyroidal extension; HR, hazard ratio; HT, Hashimoto's thyroiditis, LNM, lymph node metastasis; OR, odds ratio; PTC, papillary thyroid carcinoma, RR, risk ratio; TC, thyroid cancer.

Table 1.
Meta-analyses addressing the correlation of PTC with HT.

Jankovic et al. showed that the average prevalence rate of PTC in HT patients differed significantly between FNAB and thyroidectomy studies: 1.20 and 27.56%, respectively. Likewise, the relative risk of PTC in HT patients extended from 0.39 to 1.00 in the FNAB studies, significantly lower than that observed in the thyroidectomy studies (1.15–4.16) [37]. In that respect, Castagna et al. demonstrated absence of association of nodular HT with TC based on cytology. The same authors observed a significantly higher prevalence of DTC in nodular HT compared to nodular Graves' disease, nodular goiter with either negative or positive thyroid autoantibodies, according to surgical series. This result raised the possibility of selection bias ascribed to the fact that 60.7% of patients with nodular HT underwent surgery due to cytological data suspicious of thyroid malignancy [38]. The FNAB data from 10,508 patients revealing no statistically significant relationship between PTC and HT are consistent [104].

Nevertheless, the fear of the selection bias was abolished by the recent demonstration of a significant association of PTC with HT based on either pathological examination of surgical specimens or FNAB studies [60].

7. Effect of HT on coexistent PTC: host protective or tumor protective?

Irrespectively of whether HT is etiologically linked to PTC or merely judged "guilty by association," the importance of this coexistence lies on its clinical significance. Since a complex immune network has been considered a core component of PTC microenvironment, it is rational to assume that HT—the epitome of aberrant immune reaction—influences the progression of coexistent PTC [105]. In that respect, the positive association of a favorable outcome of coexistent PTC with HT, tumor-associated macrophage infiltration, and CD8+ lymphocytes highlights the antitumor potential of the immunological landscape intrinsic in HT [106]. The recently reported negative correlation of RORγt—a nuclear transcription protein of Th17—with lymph node metastases in PTC concurrent with HT is consistent. In fact, RORγt is positively associated with the upregulation of caveolin 1, a tumor suppressor gene [107]. Another plausible mechanism underlying the host-protective effect of HT coexistent with PTC could be the lower frequency of BRAF V600E mutation—a genetic alteration associated with aggressive PTC phenotype—in PTC concurrent with HT compared with PTC alone [41, 42].

A rich repertoire of features indicative of auspicious PTC prognosis are significantly associated with coexistent HT, including increased relapse-free and overall survival [39], increased survival rate [96, 108], decreased risk of recurrence [108], lower rate [108] or absence of extrathyroidal extension [96], and lower rate [41] or absence of lymph node metastases [96], observed in PTC coexistent with HT compared with PTC alone. The results of a recent meta-analysis including 71 published studies with 44,034 participants revealing that PTC coexistent with HT significantly correlated with reduced incidence of extrathyroidal extension, lymph node, and distant metastasis and increased recurrence-free survival duration compared with PTC alone are seminal [47]. Noticeably, the coexistence of HT with PTC has been proven an independent indicator of favorable prognosis of PTC [105], irrespectively of the extent of lymph node dissection [46], though inconsistently [108]. On the other hand, the reported absence of host-protective effect of HT on coexistent PTC [42–45] hampers the endorsement of HT as a prognostic PTC biomarker.

In fact, the inflammatory cell infiltration of tumor microenvironment plays an equivocal role, tumor-promoting versus antitumor, posing a "Dr. Jekyll or Mr. Hyde" enigma [109]. Challenging is the illumination of the precise factors that define the fate of cancer cells in the context of the interface of PTC with HT.

8. Thyroid autoantibodies in the context of HT coexistent with PTC: predictive and/or prognostic PTC biomarkers or not?

Whether HT constitutes the driving force for PTC or *vice versa* remains elusive; nevertheless, the thyroid autoantibodies, the landmark of HT, and especially the anti-thyroperoxidase autoantibodies (TPOAbs)—a more sensitive marker of HT than the TgAbs—merit interrogation as potential hallmarks of the interrelationship of PTC with HT.

A great body of evidence sustains that the positivity of thyroid autoantibodies translates into predictive and prognostic knowledge. In particular, the positivity of TPOAbs [49, 52, 53], TgAbs [51, 53, 110], as well as TPOAbs coexistent with TgAbs [52], has been shown to harbor a predictive value. Moreover, the positivity of TPOAbs [52, 57] and TgAbs [50–53, 110] has been designated as an independent predictive factor for thyroid malignancy in nodular goiter. Interestingly, the coexistence of TgAbs and TPOAbs is associated with a PTC risk greater than that connected with isolated positivity of either TgAbs or TPOAbs [52]. A host-protective role of TPOAbs in the context of coexistent PTC has been demonstrated [27, 54, 55], rationalized by the speculation that the TPOAbs exert a cytotoxic effect [110].

However, skepticism imposes a multivariate analysis failing to consolidate the host-protective effect of thyroid autoantibodies in the case of coexistent PTC [55]. Importantly, awareness raises the correlation of the positivity of thyroid autoantibodies with features indicative of ominous PTC prognosis, such as advanced disease stage [52]. As a potential link between positive thyroid autoantibodies and aggressive phenotype of PTC could be suggested the excess iodine intake that unmasks a cryptic epitope on Tg, triggering the development of TgAbs [33, 34], while exerting stimulative effect on the genesis of BRAF V600E mutation as well [111]. However, this hypothesis is debunked by the observation that the BRAF V600E mutation in DTC is inversely correlated with coexistent HT [42]. In the light of the foregoing, the designation of thyroid autoantibodies as predictive and/or prognostic biomarkers of PTC is not yet feasible.

9. Elevated TSH levels in HT coexistent with PTC: the mediator of the effect of HT on PTC?

Considering that TSH constitutes a growth factor for thyrocytes [58], rational is the designation of increased, even within the normal range, serum TSH levels, in the case of PTC concurrent with HT, as a predictor of PTC risk [49, 52, 58] and a harbinger of aggressive tumor behavior [55, 59].

A strong argument in favor of the role of TSH in thyroid tumorigenesis is the detection of activating mutations of TSH receptors (TSH-R) in DTC [112]. Moreover, the cross-talk between the TSH-R/protein kinase A (PKA) signaling transduction and the well-recognized oncogenic pathways involving Wingless/int-1 (Wnt), PI3K, and MAPK has been implicated in initiation and progression of TC [113]. However, many arguments against the pathogenetic role of TSH in TC have been raised [114–117].

Nevertheless, the demonstration of HT as a risk factor for PTC in univariate analysis while being a host-protective factor in multivariate analysis after controlling TSH levels should be mentioned [61]. Similarly, multivariate analysis showed that increased TSH levels were an independent risk factor of malignancy in most FNAB studies, albeit not consistently related to HT [60]. Consequently, the subclinical or overt hypothyroidism due to autoimmune destruction of thyroid—and not HT per se—could be the real culprit for the increased PTC risk in the context of HT.

Experimental data derived from mouse models suggest the TSH-induced signaling mediated via cyclic adenosine monophosphate (cAMP) as a prerequisite for the BRAF V600E-stimulated PTC genesis, providing a plausible explanation for the implication of elevated TSH levels in PTC [62]. Furthermore, a protein kinase C (PKC)-mediated pathway has been demonstrated in vitro to transduce the TSH-induced signaling, dictating the invasiveness and the growth of human follicular TC cell lines [118].

However, the reported association of subclinical hypothyroidism with a less aggressive PTC phenotype compared with euthyroidism cannot be ignored [119]. Consistent is the higher risk of DTC enclosed in HT requiring low levothyroxine (LT4) replacement doses as compared with HT-induced hypothyroidism requiring higher LT4 replacement doses [27]. A hypothesis mandating further exploration is that the toxic effect of TSH mediated by H_2O_2—an element essential for thyroid hormone synthesis being simultaneously a mitogenic and mutagenic factor—concerns the residual functioning thyroid tissue, while sparing the completely destructed thyroid [27].

Intriguingly, according to the European Prospective Investigation into Cancer and Nutrition (EPIC) cohort, low TSH levels may induce DTC [63], likely forming a less differentiated epithelium susceptible to malignant transformation [27]. Interestingly, two genetic variants predisposing to PTC located on 9q22.23 and 14q13.3 have been also associated with low TSH levels [120]. Consequently, the perplexing role of TSH in PTC fuels a contention regarding the endorsement of TSH levels as predictive and/or prognostic biomarker of PTC.

10. Conclusions

Despite the major strides toward the elucidation of the correlation of PTC with HT, integrating coexistent HT per se, as well as thyroid autoantibodies and TSH levels into PTC risk stratification systems, awaits further consolidation. Translating the coexistence of PTC with HT into the therapeutic approach of PTC is currently uncertain. A burning question is whether the broad clinical spectrum of HT, mirroring the wide array of HT histopathology, defines the trajectory of the coexistence of PTC with HT. The designation of HT as a premalignant lesion or PTC as a precipitating factor for HT is thwarted by the blurred, till now, pathogenetic landscape. Illuminating the temporal precedence, a parameter sine qua non for the embracement of a causal relationship between PTC and TC, is daunting. Nevertheless, harnessing the immunological link between PTC and HT should guide future efforts in clinical research, aiming to widen the horizons of immunotherapy.

In the interim, active surveillance of HT cannot be undermined, since it yields a tangible perspective of a prompt therapeutic intervention in the case of coexistent PTC.

Nonetheless, striking is, to date, the dearth of solid evidence to guide clinical decision-making on surveillance of HT based on the presumptive correlation thereof with PTC; in fact, a patient-oriented standard of care of HT should be applauded. Although thyroid ultrasonography (US) is not required for diagnosing and monitoring the majority of HT, an individualized approach should be endorsed in clinical settings. Bearing in mind the negativity of TPOAbs and/or TgAbs in 10% of HT patients [121] and approximately 20% of patients with subclinical hypothyroidism [122], identifying a hypoechoic or an inhomogeneous US thyroid pattern will provide invaluable information as regards the diagnosis of HT. Even though a thyroid/neck US is not routinely recommended unless a palpable thyroid lesion is detected [7], averting underdiagnosis of a PTC smaller than 1 centimeter (cm) in greatest dimension—the so-called papillary thyroid microcarcinoma—raises awareness. In that respect, US could unravel a nodular variant of HT that merits further evaluation. The management of nodules in the context of HT is governed by the rules applied for any thyroid nodule irrespectively of HT, based on US-guided stratification of risk of malignancy [7]. FNAB is indicated in (i) nodules equal to or larger than 1 cm in greatest dimension presenting sonographic features of high or intermediate suspicion for PTC, (ii) nodules equal to or greater than 1.5 cm in greatest dimension presenting sonographic features of low suspicion for PTC, and (iii) nodules equal to or greater than 2 cm in greatest dimension presenting features of very low suspicion for PTC. Lower size cutoffs are embraced in the presence of clinical risk factors for PTC [7]. Pending the illumination of the clinical significance of the correlation of PTC with HT, clinicians should rely on their discretion and judgment, implementing the principle "*primum non nocere*."

Conflict of interest

The authors declare no conflicts of interest.

Acronyms and abbreviations

AKT	protein kinase B
B7H1	B7 Homolog 1
cAMP	cyclic adenosine monophosphate
CCL	chemokine (C-C motif) ligand
CD	cluster of differentiation
cm	centimeter
COX-2	cyclooxygenase-2
CRI	cancer-related inflammation
CXCL	CXC chemokine ligand
CXCR4	CXC chemokine receptor 4
DCs	dendritic cells
DN	double negative
DPP IV	dipeptidyl peptidase IV
DTC	differentiated thyroid cancer
ERKs	extracellular signal-regulated kinases
FasL	Fas ligand
FNAB	fine needle aspiration biopsy
HIF-1	hypoxia-inducible factor-1
HLA	human leukocyte antigen
HLA-G	histocompatibility antigen, class 1, G, known also as human leukocyte antigen G
HT	Hashimoto's thyroiditis
IL	interleukin
iNOS	inducible nitric oxide synthases
LT4	levothyroxine
M	macrophages
MAPK	mitogen-activated protein kinase
MCP-1	monocyte chemoattractant protein 1
MMPs	matrix metalloproteinases
N	neutrophils
NK	natural killer
OPN	osteopontin

PD	programmed cell death
PD-1	PD protein 1
PD-L1	programmed cell death ligand 1
PI3K	phosphoinositide 3-kinase
PKA	protein kinase A
PKC	protein kinase C
PTC	papillary thyroid carcinoma
PTEN	phosphatase and tensin homolog
RET	rearranged during transfection
RNS	reactive nitrogen species
ROS	reactive oxygen species
TC	thyroid cancer
TgAbs	anti-thyroglobulin autoantibodies
TGFb	transforming growth factor b
Th	T-helper
TLR	Toll-like receptors
TNFa	tumor necrosis factor a
TPOAbs	anti-thyroperoxidase autoantibodies
Treg	T regulatory cells
TSH	thyroid-stimulating hormone
TSH-R	TSH receptor
UPA	urokinase-type plasminogen activator
UPAR	urokinase-type plasminogen activator receptor
US	ultrasonography
VEGF	vascular endothelial growth factor
Wnt	Wingless/int-1

Author details

Maria V. Deligiorgi* and Dimitrios T. Trafalis
Clinical Pharmacology Unit, Laboratory of Pharmacology, Medical School, National and Kapodistrian University of Athens, Athens, Greece

*Address all correspondence to: mdeligiorgi@yahoo.com

IntechOpen

© 2019 The Author(s). Licensee IntechOpen. This chapter is distributed under the terms of the Creative Commons Attribution License (http://creativecommons.org/licenses/by/3.0), which permits unrestricted use, distribution, and reproduction in any medium, provided the original work is properly cited.

References

[1] Dailey ME, Lindsay S, Skahen R. Relation of thyroid neoplasms to Hashimoto disease of the thyroid gland. AMA Archives of Surgery. 1955;**70**:291-297. DOI: 10.1001/archsurg.1955.01270080137023

[2] Coussens LM, Werb Z. Inflammation and cancer. Nature. 2002;**420**:860-867. DOI: 10.1038/nature01322

[3] Pellegriti G, Frasca F, Regalbuto C, Squatrito S, Vigneri R. Worldwide increasing incidence of thyroid cancer: Update on epidemiology and risk factors. Journal of Cancer Epidemiology. 2013;**2013**:965212. DOI: 10.1155/2013/965212

[4] Cancer Genome Atlas Research Network. Integrated genomic characterization of papillary thyroid carcinoma. Cell. 2014;**159**:676-690. DOI: 10.1016/j.cell.2014.09.050

[5] Ferlay J, Soerjomataram I, Dikshit R, Eser S, Mathers C, Rebelo M, et al. Cancer incidence and mortality worldwide: Sources, methods and major patterns in GLOBOCAN 2012. International Journal of Cancer. 2015;**136**:E359-E386. DOI: 10.1002/ijc.29210

[6] Siegel RL, Miller KD, Jemal A. Cancer statistics, 2019. CA: A Cancer Journal for Clinicians. 2019;**69**:7-34. DOI: 10.3322/caac.21551

[7] Haugen BR, Alexander EK, Bible KC, Doherty GM, Mandel SJ, Nikiforov YE, et al. 2015 American Thyroid Association Management Guidelines for Adult Patients with Thyroid Nodules and Differentiated Thyroid Cancer: The American Thyroid Association Guidelines Task Force on Thyroid Nodules and Differentiated Thyroid Cancer. Thyroid. 2016;**26**:1-133. DOI: 10.1089/thy.2015.0020

[8] Nguyen QT, Lee EJ, Huang MG, Park YI, Khullar A, Plodkowski RA. Diagnosis and treatment of patients with thyroid cancer. American Health & Drug Benefits. 2015;**8**:30-40

[9] Vigneri R, Malandrino P, Vigneri P. The changing epidemiology of thyroid cancer: Why is incidence increasing? Current Opinion in Oncology. 2015;**27**:1-7. DOI: 10.1097/CCO.0000000000000148

[10] Udelsman R, Zhang Y. The epidemic of thyroid cancer in the United States: The role of endocrinologists and ultrasounds. Thyroid. 2014;**24**:472-479. DOI: 10.1089/thy.2013.0257

[11] Morris LG, Myssiorek D. Improved detection does not fully explain the rising incidence of well-differentiated thyroid cancer: A population-based analysis. American Journal of Surgery. 2010;**200**:454-461. DOI: 10.1016/j.amjsurg.2009.11.008

[12] Wong KP, Lang BHH. The role of prophylactic central neck dissection in differentiated thyroid carcinoma: Issues and controversies. Journal of Oncology. 2011;**2011**:127929. DOI: 10.1155/2011/127929

[13] Shaha AR. Recurrent differentiated thyroid cancer. Endocrine Practice. 2012;**18**:600-603. DOI: 10.4158/EP12047.CO

[14] Qiu WH, Chen GY, Cui L, Zhang TM, Wei F, Yang Y. Identification of differential pathways in papillary thyroid carcinoma utilizing pathway co-expression analysis. Journal of BUON. 2016;**21**:1501-1509

[15] Zhao M, Wang KJ, Tan Z, Zheng CM, Liang Z, Zhao JQ. Identification of potential therapeutic targets for papillary thyroid carcinoma by bioinformatics analysis. Oncology Letters. 2016;**11**:51-58

[16] Hashimoto H. Zur Kenntis der lymphomatosen Veranderung der Schilddruse (Struma lymphomatosa). Langenbecks Archiv für klinische Chirurgie ... vereinigt mit Deutsche Zeitschrift für Chirurgie. 1912;**97**:219-248

[17] Ahmed R, Al-Shaikh S, Akhtar M. Hashimoto thyroiditis: A century later. Advances in Anatomic Pathology. 2012;**19**:181-186. DOI: 10.1097/PAP.0b013e3182534868

[18] Weetman AP. The immunopathogenesis of chronic autoimmune thyroiditis one century after Hashimoto. European Thyroid Journal. 2013;**1**:243-250. DOI: 10.1159/000343834

[19] Liu X, Zhu L, Cui D, Wang Z, Chen H, Duan Y, et al. Coexistence of histologically confirmed Hashimoto's thyroiditis with different stages of papillary thyroid carcinoma in a consecutive Chinese cohort. International Journal of Endocrinology. 2014;**2014**:769294. DOI: 10.1155/2014/769294

[20] Ward LS. Immune response in thyroid cancer: Widening the boundaries. Scientifica (Cairo). 2014;**2014**:125450. DOI: 10.1155/2014/125450

[21] Picado C, Rotter W. Precipitines seriques antithyroidiennes chez le goitreux. Comptes rendus des séances de la Société de biologie et de ses filiales. 1936;**123**:1111

[22] Rose NR, Witebsky E. Studies in organ specificity. V. Changes in the thyroid glands of rabbits following active immunization with rabbit thyroid extracts. Journal of Immunology. 1956;**76**:417-427

[23] Pyzik A, Grywalska E, Matyjaszek-Matuszek B, Roliński J. Immune disorders in Hashimoto's thyroiditis: What do we know so far? Journal of Immunology Research. 2015;**2015**:979167. DOI: 10.1155/2015/979167

[24] Li C, Yuan J, Zhu YF, Yang XJ, Wang Q, Xu J, et al. Imbalance of Th17/Treg in different subtypes of autoimmune thyroid diseases. Cellular Physiology and Biochemistry. 2016;**40**:245-252. DOI: 10.1159/000452541

[25] Stassi G, Todaro M, Bucchieri F, Stoppacciaro A, Farina F, Zummo G, et al. Fas/Fas ligand-driven T cell apoptosis as a consequence of ineffective thyroid immunoprivilege in Hashimoto's thyroiditis. Journal of Immunology. 1999;**162**:263-267

[26] Foppiani L, Secondo V, Arlandini A, Quilici P, Cabria M, Del Monte P. Thyroid lymphoma: A rare tumor requiring combined management. Hormones (Athens, Greece). 2009;**8**:214-218

[27] Paparodis R, Imam S, Todorova-Koteva K, Staii A, Jaume JC. Hashimoto's thyroiditis pathology and risk for thyroid cancer. Thyroid. 2014;**24**: 1107-1114. DOI: 10.1089/thy.2013.0588

[28] Hanahan D, Weinberg RA. Hallmarks of cancer: The next generation. Cell. 2011;**144**:646-741. DOI: 10.1016/j.cell.2011.02.013

[29] Ehlers M, Schott M. Hashimoto's thyroiditis and papillary thyroid cancer: Are they immunologically linked? Trends in Endocrinology and Metabolism. 2014;**25**:656-664. DOI: 10.1016/j.tem.2014.09.001

[30] Dong LQ, Sun XM, Xiang CF, Wu J, Yu P. Hashimoto's thyroiditis and papillary carcinoma in an adolescent girl: A case report. Molecular and Clinical Oncology. 2016;**5**:129-131. DOI: 10.3892/mco.2016.895

[31] Effraimidis G, Wiersinga WM. Mechanisms in endocrinology:

Autoimmune thyroid disease: Old and new players. European Journal of Endocrinology. 2014;**170**:R241-R252. DOI: 10.1530/EJE-14-0047

[32] Farahat SA, Mansour N, Sheta MM, Alramlawy SA, Ramadan M. Autoimmune thyroiditis among ionizing radiation exposed workers in cardiac catheterization units. Egyptian Journal of Occupational Medicine. 2017;**41**:127-1241. DOI: 10.21608/EJOM.2017.966

[33] Li Y, Teng D, Shan Z, Teng X, Guan H, Yu X, et al. Antithyroperoxidase and antithyroglobulin antibodies in a five-year follow-up survey of populations with different iodine intakes. The Journal of Clinical Endocrinology and Metabolism. 2008;**93**:1751-1757. DOI: 10.1210/jc.2007-2368

[34] Zimmermann MB, Valeria GV. Iodine intake as a risk factor for thyroid cancer: A comprehensive review of animal and human studies. Thyroid Research. 2015;**8**:8. DOI: 10.1186/s13044-015-0020-8

[35] Burstein DE, Nagi C, Wang BY, Unger P. Immunohistochemical detection of p53 homolog p63 in solid cell nests, papillary thyroid carcinoma, and Hashimoto's thyroiditis: A stem cell hypothesis of papillary carcinoma oncogenesis. Human Pathology. 2004;**35**:465-473. DOI: 10.1016/j.humpath.2003.10.027

[36] Unger P, Ewart M, Wang BY, Gan L, Kohtz DS, Burstein DE. Expression of p63 in papillary thyroid carcinoma and in Hashimoto's thyroiditis: A pathobiologic link? Human Pathology. 2003;**34**:764-769. DOI: 10.1016/S0046-8177(03)00239-9

[37] Jankovic B, Le KT, Hershman JM. Clinical review: Hashimoto's thyroiditis and papillary thyroid carcinoma: Is there a correlation? The Journal of Clinical Endocrinology and Metabolism. 2013;**98**:474-482. DOI: 10.1210/jc.2012-2978

[38] Castagna MG, Belardini V, Memmo S, Maino F, Di Santo A, Toti P, et al. Nodules in autoimmune thyroiditis are associated with increased risk of thyroid cancer in surgical series but not in cytological series: Evidence for selection bias. The Journal of Clinical Endocrinology and Metabolism. 2014;**99**:3193-3198. DOI: 10.1210/jc.2014-1302

[39] Kashima K, Yokoyama S, Noguchi S, Murakami N, Yamashita H, Watanabe S, et al. Chronic thyroiditis as a favorable prognostic factor in papillary thyroid carcinoma. Thyroid. 1998;**8**:197-202. DOI: 10.1089/thy.1998.8.197

[40] Singh B, Shaha AR, Trivedi H, Carew JF, Poluri A, Shah JP. Coexistent Hashimoto's thyroiditis with papillary thyroid carcinoma: Impact on presentation, management, and outcome. Surgery. 1999;**126**:1070-1076. DOI: 10.1067/msy.2099.101431

[41] Ma H, Li L, Li K, Wang T, Zhang Y, Zhang C, et al. Hashimoto's thyroiditis, nodular goiter or follicular adenoma combined with papillary thyroid carcinoma play protective role in patients. Neoplasma. 2018;**65**:436-440. DOI: 10.4149/neo_2018_170428N317

[42] Kim SK, Song KH, Lim SOD, Lim YC, Yoo YB, Kim JS, et al. Clinical and pathological features and the BRAF mutation in patients with papillary thyroid carcinoma with and without concurrent Hashimoto thyroiditis. Thyroid. 2009;**19**:137-141. DOI: 10.1089/thy.2008.0144

[43] Ye Z, Gu D, Hu H, Zhou Y, Hu X, Zhang X. Hashimoto's Thyroiditis, microcalcification and raised thyrotropin levels within normal range are associated with thyroid cancer. World Journal of

Surgical Oncology. 2013;**11**:56. DOI: 10.1186/1477-7819-11-56

[44] Del Rio P, Cataldo S, Sommaruga L, Concione L, Arcuri MF, Sianesi M. The association between papillary carcinoma and chronic lymphocytic thyroiditis: Does it modify the prognosis of cancer? Minerva Endocrinologica. 2008;**33**:1-5

[45] Kebebew E, Treseler PA, Ituarte PH, Clark OH. Coexisting chronic lymphocytic thyroiditis and papillary thyroid cancer revisited. World Journal of Surgery. 2001;**25**:632-637. DOI: 10.1007/s002680020165

[46] Song E, Jeon MJ, Park S, Kim M, Oh HS, Song DE, et al. Influence of coexistent Hashimoto's thyroiditis on the extent of cervical lymph node dissection and prognosis in papillary thyroid carcinoma. Clinical Endocrinology. 2018;**88**:123-128. DOI: 10.1111/cen.13475

[47] Kim SS, Lee BJ, Lee JC, Kim SJ, Jeon YK, Kim MR, et al. Coexistence of Hashimoto's thyroiditis with papillary thyroid carcinoma: The influence of central lymph node metastasis. Head & Neck. 2011;**33**:1272-1277. DOI: 10.1002/hed.21594

[48] Moon S, Chung HS, Yu JM, Yoo HJ, Park JH, Kim DS, et al. Associations between Hashimoto thyroiditis and clinical outcomes of papillary thyroid cancer: A meta-analysis of observational studies. Endocrinology and Metabolism (Seoul, Korea). 2018;**33**:473-484. DOI: 10.3803/EnM.2018.33.4.473

[49] Cho YA, Kong S-Y, Shin A, Lee J, Lee EK, Lee YJ, et al. Biomarkers of thyroid function and autoimmunity for predicting high-risk groups of thyroid cancer: A nested case–control study. BMC Cancer. 2014;**14**:873. DOI: 10.1186/1471-2407-14-873

[50] Zhang X, Zhang X, Chang Z, Wu C, Guo H. Correlation analyses of thyroid-stimulating hormone and thyroid autoantibodies with differentiated thyroid cancer. JBUON. 2018;**23**:1467-1471

[51] Kim ES, Lim DJ, Baek KH, Lee JM, Kim MK, Kwon HS, et al. Thyroglobulin antibody is associated with increased cancer risk in thyroid nodules. Thyroid. 2010;**20**:885-891. DOI: 10.1089/thy.2009.0384

[52] Wu X, Lun Y, Jiang H, Gang Q, Xin S, Duan Z, et al. Coexistence of thyroglobulin antibodies and thyroid peroxidase antibodies correlates with elevated thyroid-stimulating hormone level and advanced tumor stage of papillary thyroid cancer. Endocrine. 2013;**46**:554-560. DOI: 10.1007/s12020-013-0121-x

[53] Qin J, Yu Z, Guan H, Shi L, Liu Y, Zhao N, et al. High thyroglobulin antibody levels increase the risk of differentiated thyroid carcinoma. Disease Markers. 2015;**2015**:648670. DOI: 10.1155/2015/648670

[54] Souza SL, da Assumpção LVM, Ward LS. Impact of previous thyroid autoimmune diseases on prognosis of patients with well-differentiated thyroid cancer. Thyroid. 2003;**13**:491-495. DOI: 10.1089/105072503322021160

[55] McLeod DS, Cooper DS, Ladenson PW, Ain KB, Brierley JD, Fein HG, et al. The national thyroid cancer treatment cooperative study group. Prognosis of differentiated thyroid cancer in relation to serum thyrotropin and thyroglobulin antibody status at time of diagnosis. Thyroid. 2014;**24**:35-42. DOI: 10.1089/thy.2013.0062

[56] Morand GB, da Silva SD, Mlynarek AM, Black MJ, Payne RJ, Hier MP. Clinicopathological relevance of antithyroglobulin antibodies in low-risk papillary thyroid cancer. Clinical Otolaryngology. 2017;**42**:1130-1134. DOI: 10.1111/coa.12835

[57] Krátký J, Ježková J, Kosák M, Vítková H, Bartáková J, Mráz M, et al. Positive antithyroid antibodies and nonsuppressed TSH are associated with thyroid cancer: A retrospective cross-sectional study. International Journal of Endocrinology. 2018;**2018**:9793850. DOI: 10.1155/2018/9793850

[58] McLeod DS, Watters KF, Carpenter AD, Ladenson PW, Cooper DS, Ding EL. Thyrotropin and thyroid cancer diagnosis: A systematic review and dose-response meta-analysis. The Journal of Clinical Endocrinology and Metabolism. 2012;**97**:2682-2692. DOI: 10.1210/jc.2012-1083. Epub 2012 May 23

[59] Haymart MR, Repplinger DJ, Leverson GE, Elson DF, Sippel RS, Jaume JC, et al. Higher serum thyroid stimulating hormone level in thyroid nodule patients is associated with greater risks of differentiated thyroid cancer and advanced tumor stage. The Journal of Clinical Endocrinology and Metabolism. 2008;**93**:809-814. DOI: 10.1210/jc.2007-2215

[60] Boi F, Pani F, Mariotti S. Thyroid autoimmunity and thyroid cancer: Review focused on cytological studies. European Thyroid Journal. 2017;**6**: 1781-1786. DOI: 10.1159/000468928

[61] Zhang L, Li H, Ji QH, Zhu YX, Wang ZY, Wang Y, et al. The clinical features of papillary thyroid cancer in Hashimoto's thyroiditis patients from an area with a high prevalence of Hashimoto's disease. BMC Cancer. 2012;**12**:610. DOI: 10.1186/1471-2407-12-610

[62] Franco AT, Malaguarnera R, Refetoff S, Liao XH, Lundsmith E, Kimura S, et al. Thyrotrophin receptor signaling dependence of Braf-induced thyroid tumor initiation in mice. Proceedings of the National Academy of Sciences of the United States of America. 2011;**108**:1615-1620. DOI: 10.1073/pnas.1015557108

[63] Rinaldi S, Plummer M, Biessy C, Tsilidis KK, Østergaard JN, Overvad K, et al. Thyroid-stimulating hormone, thyroglobulin, and thyroid hormones and risk of differentiated thyroid carcinoma: The EPIC study. Journal of the National Cancer Institute. 2014;**106**:dju097. DOI: 10.1093/jnci/dju097

[64] Rahat MA, Shakya J. Parallel aspects of the microenvironment in cancer and autoimmune disease. Mediators of Inflammation. 2016;**2016**:1-17. DOI: 10.1155/2016/4375120

[65] Imam S, Dar P, Paparodis R, Almotah K, Al-Khudhair A, Hasan SA, et al. Nature of coexisting thyroid autoimmune disease determines success or failure of tumor immunity in thyroid cancer. Journal for ImmunoTherapy of Cancer. 2019;**7**:3. DOI: 10.1186/s40425-018-0483-y

[66] Harii N, Lewis CJ, Vasko V, McCall K, Benavides-Peralta U, Sun X, et al. Thyrocytes express a functional toll-like receptor 3: Overexpression can be induced by viral infection and reversed by phenylmethimazole and is associated with Hashimoto's autoimmune thyroiditis. Molecular Endocrinology. 2005;**19**:1231-1250. DOI: 10.1210/me.2004-0100

[67] McCall KD, Harii N, Lewis CJ, Malgor R, Kim WB, Saji M, et al. High basal levels of functional toll-like receptor 3 (TLR3) and noncanonical Wnt5a are expressed in papillary thyroid cancer and are coordinately decreased by phenylmethimazole together with cell proliferation and migration. Endocrinology. 2007;**148**:4226-4237. DOI: 10.1210/en.2007-0459

[68] Hajam IA, Dar PA, Shahnawaz I, Jaume JC, Lee JH. Bacterial flagellin-a potent immunomodulatory agent. Experimental & Molecular Medicine. 2017;**49**:e373. DOI: 10.1038/emm.2017.172

[69] Dvorak HF. Tumors: Wounds that do not heal-redux. Cancer Immunology Research. 2015;**3**:1-11. DOI: 10.1158/2326-6066.CIR-14-0209

[70] Imam S, Paparodis R, Sharma D, Jaume JC. Lymphocytic profiling in thyroid cancer provides clues for failure of tumor immunity. Endocrine-Related Cancer. 2014;**21**:505-516. DOI: 10.1530/ERC-13-0436

[71] Ban Y, Tozaki T, Tobe T, Ban Y, Jacobson EM, Concepcion ES, et al. The regulatory T cell gene FOXP3 and genetic susceptibility to thyroid autoimmunity: An association analysis in Caucasian and Japanese cohorts. Journal of Autoimmunity. 2007;**28**:201-207. DOI: 10.1016/j.jaut.2007.02.016

[72] Lewinski A, Sliwka PW, Stasiolek M. Dendritic cells in autoimmune disorders and cancer of the thyroid. Folia Histochemica et Cytobiologica. 2014;**52**:18-28. DOI: 10.5603/FHC.2014.0002

[73] Virchow R. Standpoints in scientific medicine, 1877. Bulletin of the History of Medicine. 1956;**30**:537-543

[74] Liotti F, Visciano C, Melillo RM. Inflammation in thyroid oncogenesis. American Journal of Cancer Research. 2012;**2**:286-297

[75] Del Prete A, Allavena P, Santoro G, Fumarulo R, Corsi MM, Mantovani A. Molecular pathways in cancer-related inflammation. Biochemia Medica. 2011;**21**:264-275

[76] Balkwill F, Charles KA, Mantovani A. Smoldering and polarized inflammation in the initiation and promotion of malignant disease. Cancer Cell. 2005;**7**:211-217. DOI: 10.1016/j.ccr.2005.02.013

[77] Kajita S, Ruebel KH, Casey MB, Nakamura N, Lloyd RV. Role of COX-2, thromboxane A2 synthase, and prostaglandin I2 synthase in papillary thyroid carcinoma growth. Modern Pathology. 2005;**18**:221-227. DOI: 10.1038/modpathol.3800285

[78] Scarpino S, Duranti E, Giglio S, Di Napoli A, Galafate D, Del Bufalo D, et al. Papillary carcinoma of the thyroid: High expression of COX-2 and low expression of KAI-1/CD82 are associated with increased tumor invasiveness. Thyroid. 2013;**23**:1127-1137. DOI: 10.1089/thy.2011.0421

[79] Nose F, Ichikawa T, Fujiwara M, Okayasu I. Up-regulation of Cyclooxygenase-2 expression in lymphocytic thyroiditis and thyroid tumors. American Journal of Clinical Pathology. 2002;**117**:546-551. DOI: 10.1309/9CCJ-XQ8P-PMFM-M65K

[80] Colotta F, Allavena P, Sica A, Garlanda C, Mantovani A. Cancer-related inflammation, the seventh hallmark of cancer: Links to genetic instability. Carcinogenesis. 2009;**30**:1073-1081. DOI: 10.1016/j.gde.2008.01.003

[81] Pozzobon T, Goldon G, Viola A, Molon B. CXCR4 signaling in health and disease. Immunology Letters. 2016;**177**:6-15. DOI: 10.1016/j.imlet.2016.06.006

[82] Larson SD, Jackson LN, Riall TS, Uchida T, Thomas RP, Qiu S, et al. Increased incidence of well-differentiated thyroid cancer associated with Hashimoto thyroiditis and the role of the PI3k/Akt pathway. Journal of the American College of Surgeons. 2007;**204**:764-773. DOI: 10.1016/j.jamcollsurg.2006.12.037

[83] Wirtschafter A, Schmidt R, Rosen D, Kundu N, Santoro M, Fusco A, et al. Expression of the RET/PTC fusion gene as a marker for papillary carcinoma in Hashimoto's thyroiditis. The Laryngoscope. 1997;**107**:95-100. DOI: 10.1097/00005537-199701000-00019

[84] Muzza M, Degl'Innocenti D, Colombo C, Perrino M, Ravasi E, Rossi S, et al. The tight relationship between papillary thyroid cancer, autoimmunity and inflammation: Clinical and molecular studies. Clinical Endocrinology. 2010;**72**:702-708. DOI: 10.1111/j.1365-2265.2009.03699.x

[85] Guarino V, Castellone MD, Avilla E, Melillo RM. Thyroid cancer and inflammation. Molecular and Cellular Endocrinology. 2010;**321**:94-102. DOI: 10.1016/j.mce.2009.10.003

[86] Kang DY, Kim KH, Kim JM, Kim SH, Kim JY, Baik HW, et al. High prevalence of RET, RAS, and ERK expression in Hashimoto's thyroiditis and in papillary thyroid carcinoma in the Korean population. Thyroid. 2007;**17**:1031-1038. DOI: 10.1089/thy.2007.0035

[87] Borrello MG, Alberti L, Fischer A, Degl'innocenti D, Ferrario C, Gariboldi M, et al. Induction of a proinflammatory program in normal human thyrocytes by the RET/PTC1 oncogene. Proceedings of the National Academy of Sciences of the United States of America. 2005;**102**:14825-14830. DOI: 10.1073/pnas.0503039102

[88] Qian F, Hanahan D, Weissman IL. L-selectin can facilitate metastasis to lymph nodes in a transgenic mouse model of carcinogenesis. Proceedings of the National Academy of Sciences of the United States of America. 2001;**98**: 3976-3981. DOI: 10.1073/pnas.061633698

[89] Castellone MD, Celetti A, Guarino V, Cirafici AM, Basolo F, Giannini R, et al. Autocrine stimulation by osteopontin plays a pivotal role in the expression of the mitogenic and invasive phenotype of RET/PTC-transformed thyroid cells. Oncogene. 2004;**23**:2188-2196. DOI: 10.1038/sj.onc.1207322

[90] Pufnock JS, Rothstein JL. Oncoprotein signaling mediates tumor-specific inflammation and enhances tumor progression. Journal of Immunology. 2009;**182**:5498-5506. DOI: 10.4049/jimmunol.0801284

[91] Gabrilovich DI, Nagaraj S. Myeloid-derived suppressor cells as regulators of the immune system. Nature Reviews. Immunology. 2009;**9**:162-174. DOI: 10.1038/nri2506

[92] Nikiforov YE. RET/PTC Rearrangement—A link between Hashimoto's thyroiditis and thyroid cancer ...or not. The Journal of Clinical Endocrinology and Metabolism. 2006;**91**:2040-2042. DOI: 10.1210/jc.2006-0791

[93] Franks AL, Slansky JE. Multiple associations between a broad spectrum of autoimmune diseases, chronic inflammatory diseases and cancer. Anticancer Research. 2012;**32**:1119-1136

[94] Girotra M, Hansen A, Farooki A, Byun DJ, Min L, Creelan BC, et al. The current understanding of the endocrine effects from immune checkpoint inhibitors and recommendations for management. JNCI Cancer Spectrum. 2018;**2**:pky021. DOI: 10.1093/jncics/pky021

[95] Zhang Y, Ma XP, Deng FS, Liu ZR, Wei HQ, Wang XH, et al. The effect of chronic lymphocytic thyroiditis on patients with thyroid cancer. World Journal of Surgical Oncology. 2014;**12**:277. DOI: 10.1186/1477-7819-12-277

[96] Lee JH, Kim Y, Choi JW, Kim YS. The association between papillary thyroid carcinoma and histologically proven Hashimoto's thyroiditis: A meta-analysis. European Journal of Endocrinology. 2013;**15**(168):343-349. DOI: 10.1530/EJE-12-0903

[97] Lai X, Xia Y, Zhang B, Li J, Jiang Y. A meta-analysis of Hashimoto's thyroiditis and papillary thyroid carcinoma risk. Oncotarget. 2017;**8**:62414-62424. DOI: 10.18632/oncotarget.18620

[98] Resende de Paiva C, Grønhøj C, Feldt-Rasmussen U, von Buchwald C. Association between Hashimoto's thyroiditis and thyroid cancer in 64,628 patients. Frontiers in Oncology. 2017;7:53. DOI: 10.3389/fonc.2017.00053

[99] McLeod DSA, Cooper DS. The incidence and prevalence of thyroid autoimmunity. Endocrine Journal. 2012;**42**:252-265

[100] Fiore E, Rago T, Scutari M, Ugolini C, Proietti A, Di Coscio G, et al. Papillary thyroid cancer, although strongly associated with lymphocytic infiltration on histology, is only weakly predicted by serum thyroid auto-antibodies in patients with nodular thyroid diseases. Journal of Endocrinological Investigation. 2009;**32**:344-335. DOI: 10.1007/BF03345725

[101] Fiore E, Latrofa F, Vitti P. Iodine, thyroid autoimmunity and cancer. European Thyroid Journal. 2015;**4**: 26-35. DOI: 10.1159/000371741

[102] Kohno Y, Yamaguchi F, Saito K, Niimi H, Nishikawa T, Hosoya T. Anti-thyroid peroxidase antibodies in sera from healthy subjects and from patients with chronic thyroiditis: Differences in the ability to inhibit thyroid peroxidase activities. Clinical and Experimental Immunology. 1991;**85**:459-463

[103] Latrofa F, Ricci D, Montanelli L, Rocchi R, Piaggi P, Sisti E, et al. Thyroglobulin autoantibodies in patients with papillary thyroid carcinoma: Comparison of different assays and evaluation of causes of discrepancies. The Journal of Clinical Endocrinology and Metabolism. 2012;**97**:3974-3982. DOI: 10.1210/jc.2012-2406

[104] Matesa-Anic D, Matesa N, Dabelic N, Kusic Z. Coexistence of papillary carcinoma and Hashimoto's thyroiditis. Acta Clinica Croatica. 2009;**48**:9-12

[105] Marotta V, Sciammarella C, Chiofalo MG, Gambardella C, Bellevicine C, Grasso M, et al. Hashimoto's thyroiditis predicts outcome in intrathyroidal papillary thyroid cancer. Endocrine-Related Cancer. 2017;**24**:485-493. DOI: 10.1530/ERC-17-0085

[106] Cunha LL, Morari EC, Guihen AC, Razolli D, Gerhard R, Nonogaki S, et al. Infiltration of a mixture of immune cells may be related to good prognosis in patients with differentiated thyroid carcinoma. Clinical Endocrinology. 2012;**77**:918-925. DOI: 10.1111/j.1365-2265.2012.04482.x

[107] Zeng R, Lyu Y, Zhang G, et al. Positive effect of RORγt on the prognosis of thyroid papillary carcinoma patients combined with Hashimoto's thyroiditis. American Journal of Translational Research. 2018;**10**:3011-3024

[108] Jeong JS, Kim HK, Lee CR, Park S, Park JH, Kang SW, et al. Coexistence of chronic lymphocytic thyroiditis with papillary thyroid carcinoma: Clinical manifestation and prognostic outcome. Journal of Korean Medical Science. 2012;**27**:883-889. DOI: 10.3346/jkms.2012.27.8.883

[109] Talmadge JE, Donkor M, Scholar E. Inflammatory cell infiltration of tumors: Jekyll or Hyde. Cancer Metastasis Reviews. 2007;**26**:373-400. DOI: 10.1007/s10555-007-9072-0

[110] Azizi G, Keller JM, Lewis M, et al. Association of Hashimoto's thyroiditis with thyroid cancer. Endocrine-Related Cancer. 2014;**21**:845-852. DOI: 10.1530/ERC-14-0258

[111] Kim HJ, Park HK, Byun DW, Suh K, Yoo MH, Min YK, et al. Iodine intake

as a risk factor for BRAF mutations in papillary thyroid cancer patients from an iodine-replete area. European Journal of Nutrition. 2018;**57**:809-815. DOI: 10.1007/s00394-016-1370-2

[112] Russo D, Arturi F, Chiefari E, Filetti S. Thyrotropin receptor: A role for thyroid tumourigenesis? Forum (Genoa, Italy). 1999;**9**(2):166-175

[113] García-Jiménez C, Santisteban P. TSH signalling and cancer. Arquivos Brasileiros de Endocrinologia e Metabologia. 2007;**51**(5):654-671

[114] Matsuo K, Friedman E, Gejman PV, Fagin JA. The thyrotropin receptor (TSH-R) is not an oncogene for thyroid tumors: Structural studies of the TSH-R and the α-subunit of Gs in human thyroid neoplasms. The Journal of Clinical Endocrinology and Metabolism. 1993;**76**:1446-1451. DOI: 10.1210/jcem.76.6.8501149

[115] Derwahl M, Broecker M, Kraiem Z. Thyrotropin may not be the dominant growth factor in benign and malignant thyroid tumors. The Journal of Clinical Endocrinology and Metabolism. 1998;**84**:829-834. DOI: 10.1210/jcem.84.3.5519

[116] Shi Y, Zou M, Farid NR. Expression of thyrotropin receptor gene in thyroid carcinoma is associated with good prognosis. Clinical Endocrinology. 1993;**39**:269-274

[117] Satta MA, DeRosa G, Testa A, Maussier ML, Valenza V, Rabitti C, et al. Thyroid cancer in suppressed contralateral lobe of patients with hot thyroid nodule. European Journal of Cancer. 1993;**29A**:1190-1192

[118] Hoelting T, Tezelman S, Siperstein AE, Duh QY, Clark OH. Thyrotropin stimulates invasion and growth of follicular thyroid cancer cells via PKC- rather than PKA-activation. Biochemical and Biophysical Research Communications. 1993;**195**:1230-1236. DOI: 10.1006/bbrc.1993.2176

[119] Ahn D, Sohn JH, Kim JH, Shin CM, Jeon JH, Park JY. Preoperative subclinical hypothyroidism in patients with papillary thyroid carcinoma. American Journal of Otolaryngology. 2013;**34**:312-319. DOI: 10.1016/j.amjoto.2012.12.013. Epub 2013 Jan 26

[120] Gudmundsson J, Sulem P, Gudbjartsson DF, Jonasoon JG, Sigurdsson A, Bergthorsson JT, et al. Common variants on 9q22.33 and 14q13.3 predispose to thyroid cancer in European populations. Nature Genetics. 2009;**41**:460-464. DOI: 10.1038/ng.339

[121] Mincer DL, Jialal I. Hashimoto thyroiditis. In: StatPearls [Internet]. Treasure Island (FL): StatPearls Publishing; 2018

[122] Pearce SH, Brabant G, Duntas LH, Monzani F, Peeters RP, Razvi S, et al. 2013 ETA guideline: Management of subclinical hypothyroidism. European Thyroid Journal. 2013;**2**:215-228

Chapter 5

Thyroid Cancer and Acromegaly

Carla Souza Pereira Sobral, Marcelo Magalhães and Manuel dos Santos Faria

Abstract

Acromegaly results from oversecretion of growth hormone and subsequent insulin growth factor-I. Some studies have described an association between acromegaly and increased risk of some cancers, including thyroid cancer, the most common endocrine malignancy. It is well known that follicular thyroid cells express IGF-I receptor and that GH and IGF-I have both proliferative and anti-apoptotic effects and their hypersecretion may theoretically induce tumor development and stimulate its growth, despite the fact that research data is conflicting and population-based data on thyroid cancer and acromegaly is rare. Some molecular alterations, including point mutations in *BRAF* and *RAS* genes and *RET/PTC* gene rearrangements, have been associated with oncogenesis of PTC. However, the implications of these genetic markers in the development of PTC in patients with acromegaly are not yet well known. In this chapter, we discuss epidemiology, pathogenesis, molecular biology aspects, and how to screen and to manage acromegalic patients with nodular thyroid disease and thyroid cancer.

Keywords: acromegaly and thyroid cancer, IGF-I and cancer, thyroid and acromegaly, GH and cancer, molecular markers and thyroid cancer

1. Introduction

Acromegaly is a rare disease that results from the oversecretion of growth hormone (GH) and subsequent insulin growth factor I (IGF-I) [1]. It is associated with important complications that may reduce life expectancy of these patients [2, 3].

Most acromegalic patients die from cardiovascular, cerebrovascular, or respiratory diseases [3, 4]. Nevertheless, in the past two decades, some studies have also described an association between acromegaly and an increased risk of some cancers such as colorectal and thyroid cancer (TC), which is the most common endocrine malignancy, among others [5].

Part of the difficulty in determining the true incidence of cancer in this population is due to the relative rarity of acromegaly [6]. On the other hand, with improvement in surgical and radiotherapeutic procedures as well as advances in medical treatment, an increase of the survival rate of patients with acromegaly has been shown. As a result, patients may have a longer exposure to high GH levels [7].

As the prevalence of thyroid cancer has been shown to increase among patients with acromegaly, this should draw attention for clinicians to investigate thyroid disease, particularly thyroid cancer.

2. Epidemiology

The association between acromegaly and TC is supported by preclinical data showing that GH-IGF system plays an important role in cancer development and progression [6]. However, clinical studies that addressed the association between acromegaly and cancer produced controversial results, partly due to the different methodological approaches used (case-control and population-based designs) [8].

A comprehensive meta-analysis showed an increased risk of both nodular thyroid disease (NTD) (OR = 6.9, RR = 2.1) and TC (OR = 7.5, RR = 7.2) in acromegaly. It showed a prevalence slightly below 60% of NTD and of around 4% of TC [8]. Within this context, a consistent Brazilian multicentric study with 124 acromegalic patients in a case-control design showed a higher prevalence of 7.2% for TC and 0.7% in the control group [9].

These findings may result from the fact of improving diagnostic and treatment of acromegaly extending the life duration which increases the prevalence of both benign and malignant neoplasms [3–11].

On the other hand, the co-occurrence of autoimmune thyroid diseases and acromegaly is not common. So far only a handful of cases of Graves-Basedow disease in acromegalic patients have been reported, while Hashimoto's disease occurs more frequently (4.6%) [12, 13].

3. Molecular pathogenesis of TC in acromegalic patients

3.1 Molecular basis of acromegaly

The pituitary gland integrates hormonal signs that control several homeostatic processes such as metabolism, growth, and reproduction. Cell clusters localized in the anterior pituitary, somatotrophs, secrete GH responsible for cellular proliferation through membrane-bound growth hormone receptor (GHR) present in various organs and systems [14]. The interaction between GH and GHR results in activation of intracellular protein Janus kinase 2 (JAK2). As shown in **Figure 1**, once phosphorylated JAK2 activates the signal transducers and activators of transcription (STAT) protein that is translocated to the nucleus and initiates transcription of genes in response to GH [15], the STAT is able to bind to IGF-I promoter regulating the transcription of this gene [16]. Thus, the presence of GH can induce the synthesis of IGF-I that occurs mainly in the liver and is composed of 70 amino acids and has mitotic and anti-apoptotic effects [1].

In the vast majority of cases, the excess of GH in acromegaly is originated from proliferating somatotrophs (somatotropinoma). The pituitary adenomas are of monoclonal origin, indicating that the tumor rises from a single cell that acquires proliferative advantage [17]. The primary defect that leads to development of somatotropinoma may result from genetic and epigenetic alterations inducing the activation of oncogenes or inactivation of tumor suppressor genes [1]. Mutations in the alpha subunit of transmembrane G protein is observed in 40% of GH-secreting tumors [1]. This abnormality may cause constitutive activation of cyclin AMP (cAMP) and consequent hypersecretion of GH. Loss of expression of proapoptotic molecules such as GADD45γ (growth arrest and DNA damage-inducible 45γ protein) and overexpression of oncoproteins, including PTTG (pituitary tumor-transforming gene), are phenomena also observed in pituitary adenomas [17, 18].

Most cases of acromegaly occur sporadically; however, approximately 5% of cases may be related to inherited diseases such as multiple endocrine neoplasia type 1 (MEN1), Carney complex (CNC), and familial isolated pituitary adenoma

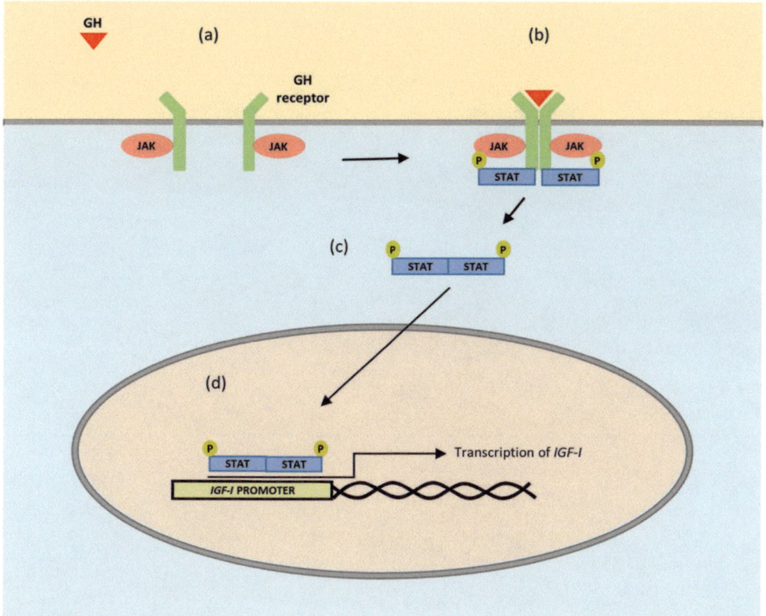

Figure 1.
Activation of JAK/STAT pathway mediated by GH (growth hormone). (a) JAK/STAT pathway components are inactive. (b) GH leads to dimerization of its receptor promoting phosphorylation of JAK and consequent activation of STAT proteins. (c) Once activated, STAT forms dimers that are translocated to the cell nucleus. (d) The STAT dimers in the nucleus are capable of binding to IGF-I promoter, initiating the transcription of this gene.

(FIPA) [17]. Germline mutations in aryl hydrocarbon receptor-interacting protein (*AIP*) gene seem to be the most frequent genetic alteration detected in sporadic and familial acromegaly patients [19]. The MEN1 and CNC are caused mainly by defects in genes *MEN1* (menin) and *PRKAR1A* (regulatory subunit type 1 alpha), respectively [17].

3.2 Cross talk between acromegaly and thyroid cancer

The serum GH excess may promote proliferation and suppress apoptosis in many tissues [15]. Thus, it is suggested that acromegaly is responsible for the increased risk for development of many malignancies. PTC is the most common thyroid cancer observed in acromegaly [7, 9]. This type of pituitary tumor can also be associated with benign thyroid conditions such as diffuse and nodular goiters [9].

The mechanism of thyroid carcinogenesis in acromegaly is attributed to an autocrine/paracrine loop for GH/IGF-I in tumor tissue [8]. As the thyroid follicular cells also produce IGF-I and express genes encoding IGF-IR, the long-term exposure of thyrocyte to high GH/IGF-I levels may work synergically with this loop in promoting goiter development and malignant transformation [20].

3.3 Molecular mechanisms and potential biomarkers of thyroid carcinogenesis in acromegaly

As shown in **Figure 2**, the molecular oncogenesis of PTC is mainly related to deregulation of mitogen-activated protein kinase (MAPK) signaling pathway and involves point mutations in *BRAF* and *RAS* genes and *RET/PTC* gene rearrangements [21, 22]. Analysis of these molecular markers can have diagnostic and prognostic implications in thyroid cancer.

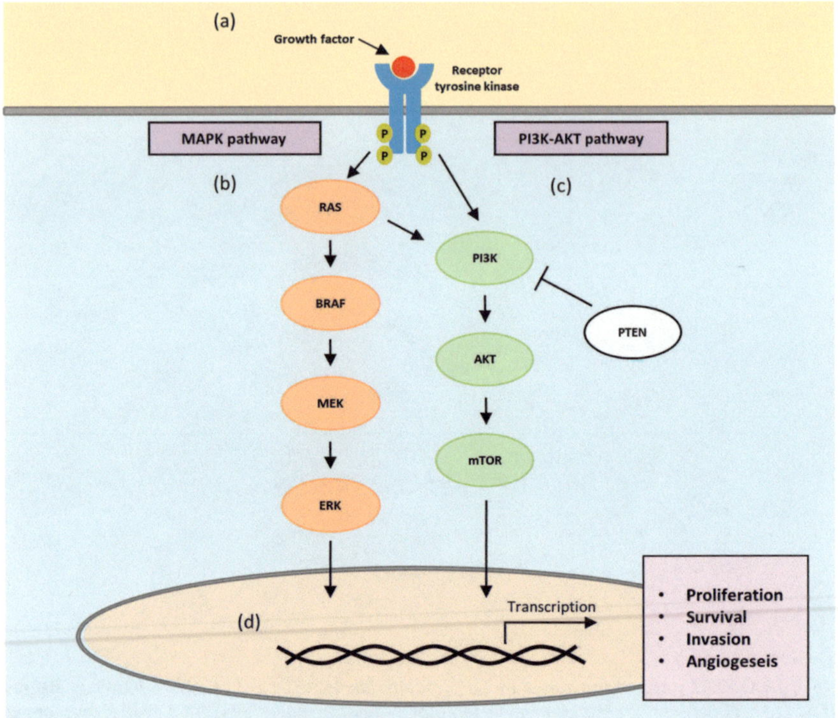

Figure 2.
MAPK and PI3K pathways. (a) Growth factors bind to receptor tyrosine kinase and trigger the activation of (b) MAPK and/or (c) PI3K-AKT. (d) The signaling mediated to both pathways promotes the transcription of gene associated to different cellular processes such as proliferation and survival.

3.3.1 BRAF mutation

BRAF (B-type RAF kinase) is a serine threonine kinase considered the most potent MAPK activator. This protein regulates important cellular processes such as proliferation, differentiation, and apoptosis [1].

In PTC, the main mechanism for activation of *BRAF* gene is a point mutation that promotes a substitution of nucleotide thymine by adenine at position 1799. This single nucleotide change promotes the replacement of valine by glutamate at protein residue 600 (V600E). The *BRAF* V600E mutation is the most frequent genetic abnormality reported in thyroid carcinomas in the general population, particularly in PTC [21].

In acromegalic patients, the importance of *BRAF* V600E mutation on PTC carcinogenesis is still not well defined. In an Italian cohort of acromegalic patients, the *BRAF* V600E mutation was detected in 70% of cases with PTC, suggesting that this mutation is the main genetic driver of neoplastic transformation of thyroid cells in acromegaly [23]. On the other hand, other studies have demonstrated that the *BRAF* V600E mutation is infrequent in patients PTC with and without acromegaly [20, 24]. In these reports lower prevalence of this genetic alteration in acromegalic patients with PTC than non-acromegalic cases with PTC was verified. These results suggest that *BRAF* V600E mutation may not be a main mechanism of malignant transformation of thyroid cells in patients with acromegaly.

3.3.2 RAS mutations

The *HRAS*, *KRAS*, and *NRAS* are homologous gene members of the *RAS* (retrovirus-associated DNA sequences) family. These genes encode GTP-binding proteins localized at the inner superficial of the cell membrane involved in signaling MAPK and PI3K-AKT pathways [1]. Together, *RAS* mutations are the second most frequent molecular alteration found in thyroid cancer, occurring in 10–20% of PTC cases and 40–50% of follicular carcinomas [22].

Point mutations are commonly restricted at codon 61 of the *HRAS* and *NRAS* genes and at codons 12 and 13 in the *KRAS* gene. *RAS* mutations in thyroid cancer have been associated to favorable prognosis such as tumor encapsulation and absence of metastases but also may represent a poor prognostic factor predisposing to cellular dedifferentiation and anaplastic transformation [22]. *NRAS* codon 61 mutation has been referred as the most frequent genetic alteration in PTC patients with acromegaly. Aydin et al. pointed out that patients with *NRAS* codon 61 mutation have aggressive histologic features such as vascular and capsular invasion [24]. However, another study revealed no case in a cohort of acromegalic patients with PTC-harbored *RAS* mutations [23]. These contradictory findings indicate that the importance of *RAS* mutational status in thyroid oncogenesis in acromegaly remains to be clarified.

3.3.3 RET/PTC rearrangements

The *RET* is a proto-oncogene that encodes a receptor-type tyrosine kinase with three domains: extracellular, transmembrane, and intracellular tyrosine kinase. The activation of this gene can contribute to the development of several neoplasms [25]. Rearrangements of *RET* that originated from fusion with unrelated genes (RET/PTC rearrangements) have been reported in thyroid follicular cells [26]. This genomic alteration can produce a chimeric oncoprotein with inappropriate tyrosine kinase activity able to continually stimulate the MAPK and PI3K-AKT pathways [26]. Among the fusion variants of *RET*, the rearrangements RET/PTC1 and RET/PTC3 are the most frequent in thyroid cancer. Whereas in RET/PTC1 the *RET* gene is fused to *CCDC6* (known as *H4*), in RET/PTC3 the rearrangement occurs with *NCOA4* (known as *ELE1* or *RFG*) [25]. RET/PTC rearrangement appears to be an important mechanism of thyroid carcinogenesis, but its frequency has oscillated in different reports. This genetic abnormality was not detected in PTC patients with acromegaly [24], although studies with this approach are rare in acromegaly.

3.3.4 Other molecular alterations

Besides the potential classic marker, other molecules have been evaluated in relation to their implication on PTC development in acromegaly, among them are IGF-I, IGF-IRβ, AIP, AHR, and galectin-3 (Gal-3) [20, 23–24, 27].

The analysis of immunohistochemical staining for IGF-IRβ revealed a high expression of this receptor in PTC samples [20]. Although differences in IGF-IRβ tumoral staining between PTC patients with and without acromegaly have not been observed, this marker had significantly less expression in adjacent normal tissue of patients with acromegaly. These data suggest that high GH levels may trigger autocrine and paracrine effects of IGF-I in thyroid follicular cells resulting in overexpression of IGF-IRβ in tumor tissue of acromegalic patients. In line with these results, it was observed that PTC patients with acromegaly have higher expression of IGF-I than PTC cases without acromegaly [27]. Additionally, an intense expression was verified of Gal-3 in PTC with acromegaly, speculating a possible influence of this protein on thyroid carcinogenesis.

As previously mentioned, inactivation of *AIP* gene is frequently reported in pituitary tumors. However, this genetic abnormality seems not to be determinant to thyroid carcinogenesis in acromegalic patients [23]. Furthermore, there are no differences in AIP protein expression between PTC in patients with and without acromegaly. Although immunohistochemical analysis for AIP receptor (AHR) has shown strong staining of PTC samples carrying *BRAF* V600E compared with wild type, differences were not found in AHR staining between PTC in acromegalic and non-acromegalic patients [23]. Thus, molecular alterations in AIP and AHR cannot be related to PTC carcinogenesis in acromegaly.

4. How to screen NTD in acromegalic patients

NTD seems to be significantly more frequent in patients with acromegaly. Even palpable thyroid nodules occur significantly more often in these patients [9, 13].

Periodic thyroid ultrasound (US) and careful evaluation of detected lesions are important parts in the follow-up of acromegalic patients. The sonographic characteristics considered to be suspicious of TC, such as microcalcifications, irregular margins (infiltrative and microlobulated), taller than wide shape, and rim calcifications with small extrusive soft tissue component (evidence of extrathyroidal extension), are the same of the general population with NTD [5, 9].

Fine-needle aspiration (FNA) is the procedure of choice in the evaluation on NTD, and it should be performed when clinically indicated according to nodule's size and US appearance. The FNA cytology result must be reported using the Bethesda System for Reporting Thyroid Cytopathology [9, 28].

In summary, as the risk of malignancy in thyroid nodules in these patients is about 8%, which is in the range considered for the general population, the management of NTD should follow the current guidelines [9, 28].

5. How to treat TC in acromegalic patients

Although there is a risk of TC in acromegalic patients, its clinical behavior does not seem to be different [5]. Therefore, acromegalic patients with TC may be treated with total thyroidectomy or hemithyroidectomy according to its FNA result and size and the presence of clinically apparent metastatic lymph nodes [28].

Before surgery, we suggest that all acromegalic patients should do a preoperative voice assessment (preoperative laryngeal exam—laryngoscopy) because they frequently have soft tissue thickening and edema of the tongue, pharynx, and upper airways [3]. Also, they must have a careful evaluation of comorbidities as hypertension, diabetes mellitus, and cardiovascular disease [3].

After surgery, these patients may or may not receive radioiodine depending, if it is a differentiated TC, on its risk of recurrence [28]. Studies about the relationship between medullary thyroid cancer (MTC) and acromegaly are lacking.

The frequency of US and laboratory tests during TC follow-up should follow the current guidelines.

6. Conclusion

NTC and TC are more frequent in acromegalic patients. On the other hand, the studies about potential mechanisms involved in this association between TC and acromegaly are still scarce, and besides they include small sample sizes. Furthermore, in these few reports, there is no marker clearly implicated on diagnosis or prognosis of PTC. Thus, further studies with this approach are needed.

We suggest that acromegalic patients should be routinely screened by thyroid ultrasound and during their follow-up as necessary. Its management should follow the current guidelines. This is very important because it may allow early diagnosis and treatment of TC.

Acknowledgements

We would like to thank Doctor Gilvan Nascimento Cortês for the review of the manuscript.

Conflict of interest

There is no conflict of interest.

Author details

Carla Souza Pereira Sobral[1,3], Marcelo Magalhães[1,2,3]
and Manuel dos Santos Faria[1,2,3*]

1 Endocrinology Unit, University Hospital of the Federal University of Maranhão (HUUFMA), Brazil

2 Clinical Research Center of the University Hospital of the Federal University of Maranhão, Brazil (CEPEC—HUUFMA), Brazil

3 Research Group in Clinical and Molecular Endocrinology and Metabology (ENDOCLIM—HUUFMA), Brazil

*Address all correspondence to: mfaria@inlabmail.com

IntechOpen

© 2019 The Author(s). Licensee IntechOpen. This chapter is distributed under the terms of the Creative Commons Attribution License (http://creativecommons.org/licenses/by/3.0), which permits unrestricted use, distribution, and reproduction in any medium, provided the original work is properly cited.

References

[1] Melmed S. Acromegaly pathogenesis and treatment. Journal of Clinical Investigation. 2009;**119**:3189-3202. DOI: 10.1172/JCI39375

[2] Holdaway IM, Rajasoorya RC, Gamble GD. Factors influencing mortality in acromegaly. Journal of Clinical Endocrinology and Metabolism. 2004;**89**:667-674. DOI: 10.1210/jc.2003-031199

[3] Katznelson L, Laws ER Jr, Melmed S. Acromegaly: An endocrine society clinical practice guideline. Journal of Clinical Endocrinology and Metabolism. 2014;**99**:3933-3951. DOI: 10.1210/jc.2014-2700

[4] Arosio M, Reimondo G, Malchiodi E. Predictors of morbidity and mortality in acromegaly: An Italian survey. European Journal of Endocrinology. 2012;**167**:189-198. DOI: 10.1530/EJE-12-0084

[5] Terzolo M, Reimondo G, Berchialla P. Acromegaly is associated with increased cancer risk: A survey in Italy. Endocrine-Related Cancer. 2017;**24**:495-504. DOI: 10.1530/ERC-16-0553

[6] Wolinski K, Czarnywojtek A, Ruchala M. Risk of thyroid nodular disease and thyroid cancer in patients with acromegaly—Meta-analysis and systematic review. PLoS One. 2014;**9**:e8878. DOI: 10.1371/journal.pone.0088787

[7] Reverter JL, Fajardo C, Resmini E. Benign and malignant nodular thyroid disease in acromegaly. Is a routine thyroid ultrasound evaluation advisable? PLoS One. 2014;**9**:e104174. DOI: 10.1371/journal.pone.0104174

[8] Loeper S, Ezzat S. Acromegaly: Re-thinking the cancer risk. Reviews in Endocrine and Metabolic Disorders. 2008;**9**:41-58. DOI: 10.1007/s11154-007-9063-z

[9] Santos MC, Nascimento GC, Nascimento AG. Thyroid cancer in patients with acromegaly: A case–control study. Pituitary. 2013;**16**:109-114. DOI: 10.1007/s11102-012-0383-y

[10] Boguszewski CL, Ayuk J. Management of endocrine disease: Acromegaly and cancer risk: An old debate revisited. European Journal of Endocrinology. 2016;**175**:147-156. DOI: 10.1530/EJE-16-0178

[11] Maione L, Brue T, Beckers A. Changes in the management and comorbidities of acromegaly over three decades: The French Acromegaly Registry. European Journal of Endocrinology. 2017;**176**:645-655. DOI: 10.1530/EJE-16-1064

[12] Xia W, Gao L, Guo X. GH, IGF-1, and age are important contributors to thyroid abnormalities in patients with acromegaly. International Journal of Endocrinology. 2018;**2018**:6546832. DOI: 10.1155/2018/6546832

[13] Wüster C, Steger G, Schmelzle A.Increased incidence of euthyroid and hyper-thyroid GO iters in dependently of thyrotropin in patients with acromegaly. Hormone and Metabolic Research. 1991;**23**:131-134. DOI: 10.1055/s-2007-1003632

[14] Nathan J, Lanning CC. Recent advances in growth hormone signaling. Reviews in Endocrine & Metabolic Disorders. 2006;7:225-223. DOI: 10.1007/s11154-007-9025-5

[15] Loeper S, Ezzat S. Acromegaly: Re-thinking the cancer risk. Reviews in Endocrine & Metabolic Disorders. 2008;**9**:41-58. DOI: 10.1007/s11154-007-9063-z

[16] Chia DJ, Ono M, Woelfle J. Characterization of distinct Stat5b binding sites that mediate growth hormone-stimulated IGF-I gene transcription. Journal of Biological Chemistry. 2006;**6**:3190-3197. DOI: 10.1074/jbc.M510204200

[17] Horvath A, Constantine A. Stratakis: Clinical and molecular genetics of acromegaly: MEN1, Carney complex, McCune-Albright syndrome, familial acromegaly and genetic defects in sporadic tumors. Reviews in Endocrine & Metabolic Disorders. 2008;**9**:1-11. DOI: 10.1007/s11154-007-9066-9

[18] Melmed S. Acromegaly: Review article. The New England Journal of Medicine. 2006;**355**:2558-2573

[19] Vierimaa O, Georgitsi M, Lehtonen R. Pituitary adenoma predisposition caused by germline mutations in the AIP gene. Science. 2006;**312**:1228. DOI: 10.1126/science.1126100

[20] Kim HK, Lee JS, Park MH. Tumorigenesis of papillary thyroid cancer is not BRAF-dependent in patients with acromegaly. PLoS One. 2014;**10**:e110241. DOI: 10.1371/journal.pone.0110241

[21] Kimura ET, Nikiforova MN, Zhaowen Z. High prevalence of BRAF mutations in thyroid cancer: Genetic evidence for constitutive activation of the RET/PTC-RAS-BRAF signaling pathway in papillary thyroid carcinoma. Cancer Research. 2003;**63**:1454-1457

[22] Koster EJ, Geus-Oei LF, Dekkers OM. Diagnostic utility of molecular and imaging biomarkers in cytological indeterminate thyroid nodules. Endocrine Reviews. 2018;**39**:154-191. DOI: 10.1210/er.2017-00133

[23] Mian C, Ceccato F, Barollo S. AHR over-expression in papillary thyroid carcinoma: Clinical and molecular assessments in a series of italian acromegalic patients with a long-term follow-up. PLoS One. 2014;**7**:e101560. DOI: 10.1371/journal.pone.0101560

[24] Aydin K, Aydin C, Dagdelen S. Genetic alterations in differentiated thyroid cancer patients with acromegaly. Experimental and Clinical Endocrinology & Diabetes. 2015;**124**:198-202. DOI: 10.1055/s-0035-1565061

[25] Mulligan LM. RET revisited: Expanding the oncogenic portfolio. Nature Reviews Cancer. 2014;**14**: 173-186. DOI: 10.1038/nrc3680

[26] Nikiforov YE, Nikiforova MN. Molecular genetics and diagnosis of thyroid cancer. Focus on Thyroid Cancer. 2011;**7**:569-580. DOI: 10.1038/nrendo.2011.142

[27] Keskin FE, Ozkaya HM, Ferahman S. The role of different molecular markers in papillary thyroid cancer patients with acromegaly. Experimental and Clinical Endocrinology & Diabetes. 2018. DOI: 10.1055/a-0629-9223

[28] Bruchim I, Attias Z, Werner H. Targeting the IGF1 axis in cancer proliferation. Expert Opinion on Therapeutic Targets. 2009;**13**:1179-1181. DOI: 10.1517/14728220903201702

Chapter 6

Intraoperative Neuromonitoring in Thyroid Surgery

Fabio Medas, Gian Luigi Canu, Enrico Erdas and Pietro Giorgio

Abstract

Recurrent laryngeal nerve (RLN) injury is the most feared complication in thyroid surgery, resulting in a worse patients' quality of life, and is the most common cause of medical claim. Visualization of RLN before proceeding with dissection of the gland is considered the gold standard. In the last decade, intraoperative neuromonitoring (IONM) of RLN has progressively gained acceptance; nowadays, this method is widely spread, being routinely used in large workflow centers. IONM is helpful in the identification of RLN and allows to asses nerve functionality during and at the end of surgical procedure. In this chapter, IONM features, its advantages and limits, and its usefulness will be discussed.

Keywords: thyroid surgery, thyroid carcinoma, intraoperative neuromonitoring, recurrent laryngeal nerve, nerve injury

1. Introduction

Postoperative recurrent laryngeal nerve (RLN) injury is one of the most feared complications during thyroid surgery. Even in experienced hands, transient RLN palsy occurs in 0.4–12% of cases [1–3], while permanent palsy is reported in up to 5–6% [2, 4]; its frequency is lower (0.2–0.8%) in hospitals with a large workflow [5]. RLN palsy can significantly deteriorate patients' quality of life, causing hoarseness of voice, dysphonia and dysphagia. Bilateral RLN palsy is an uncommon but life-threatening complication, even if transient, since it is associated to airway obstruction, which is potentially lethal for the patient. Intraoperative RLN injuries are due to transection and traction of the nerve, electrical and thermal injuries, suture entrapment and excessive skeletization. The risk of nerve palsy increases during surgery for thyroid cancer, especially in case of large or locally advanced tumors that can dislocate or infiltrate the nerve, during central compartment lymph node dissection (CLND) or in case of revision surgery. Over the years, surgical approach to RLN has consistently changed: the first approach, consisting in non-visualization and avoidance of the nerve, has been replaced with routine identification of RLN, which has been reported to be associated with a lower incidence of RLN palsy [6–10].

Intraoperative neuromonitoring (IONM) of RNL during thyroid surgery has widely spread during the last decade as an adjunct to the gold standard of direct visualization of the nerve; nowadays, it has become standard practice in thyroid surgery for many surgeons [11]. The most common method currently in use for

RLN monitoring is an endotracheal tube containing electrodes embedded on it, placed in close proximity to vocal cords, that register effects of stimulation of RLN. IONM is able to detect anatomic variations of the nerve and to clarify the mechanism and the site of the injury, and to predict vocal cord function after surgery. During surgical procedure, repeated tissue stimulation is helpful to correctly identify the nerve. Furthermore, IONM can detect non-function nerves that appear anatomically intact.

2. Intraoperative neuromonitoring in thyroid surgery

Intraoperative neuromonitoring has been introduced in thyroid surgery as an adjunct to standard visual identification of the recurrent laryngeal nerve (RLN) to prevent nerve lesion. The use of IONM, besides helping to identify the RLN, gives an objective evaluation of its function during the whole dissection [12–15]. IONM was introduced about 50 years ago, and various neuromonitoring methods (glottic pressure method, glottic monitoring method, insertion of needle electrodes in vocal cords endoscopically or through cricothyroid membrane, laryngeal palpation method, and monitoring via endotracheal tube with surface electrodes) have been utilized [16]. For several reasons, such as simplicity, non-invasiveness, and safety, IONM via endotracheal (ET) tube with surface electrodes has become the standard method [12]. It consists in an electromyography (EMG) that evaluates the vocal cord adductor function by using surface electrodes on the ET tube. NIM-Response 3.0 System (Medtronic Xomed, Jacksonville, Florida, USA) is the most widely used device for RLN monitoring (**Figure 1**). It transforms laryngeal muscle activity into audible and visual EMG signals whenever the RLN or vagus nerve is stimulated intraoperatively. This system basically consists of the combination of two electrical circuits: stimulation and recording sides. The stimulation side consists of a stimulator probe (nerve stimulator probe, continuous vagus nerve stimulator probe), which transmits electric current to the nerve, and a grounding electrode. The nerve stimulation probe can be monopolar or bipolar, while the continuous monitoring probes applied to the vagus nerve can be monopolar, bipolar, or tripolar. The

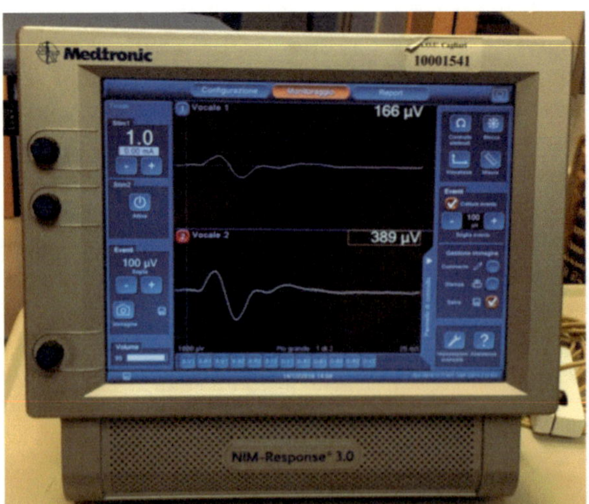

Figure 1.
NIM-Response 3.0 System (Medtronic Xomed, Jacksonville, Florida, USA) (Italian configuration). In thyroid surgery, two channels for the right and left vocal cords are sufficient and 2 EMG screens appear on the monitor.

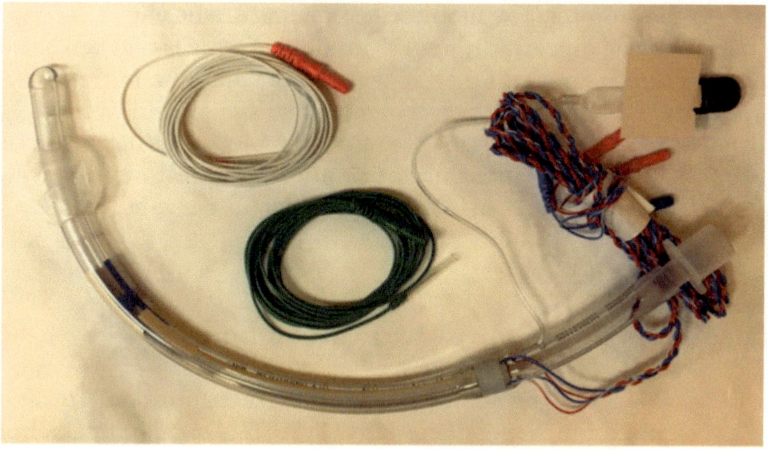

Figure 2.
ET tube with surface electrodes and grounding electrodes (white: stimulation side, green: recording side).

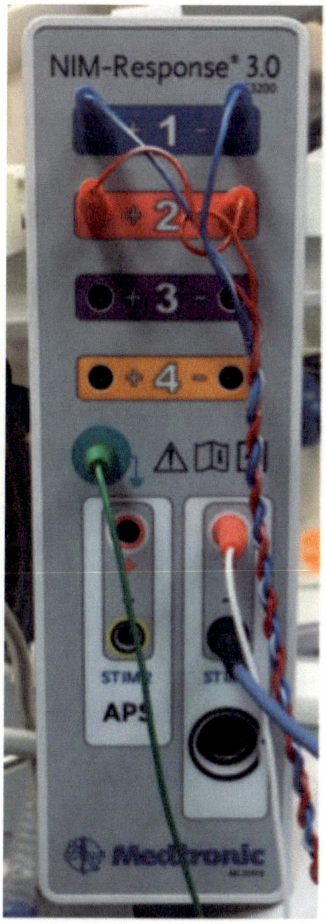

Figure 3.
Stimulation and recording sides are combined on the interconnect box, through which they connect to the monitor.

recording side, instead, consists of the ET tube with surface electrodes, which are placed at the level of the vocal cord, and their ground electrode (**Figure 2**). These two main systems combine on the interconnection box (**Figure 3**), through which they connect to the monitor. The monitoring systems can be with 2, 4, 8, or 16 channels. The number of channels indicates the number of nerves that can be monitored. A separate EMG screen appears for each nerve on the monitor. In thyroid surgery, two channels for the right and left vocal cords are sufficient and two EMG screens appear on the monitor (**Figure 1**). In case of continuous vagus nerve stimulation, instead, two EMG screens for intermittent monitoring appear on the left side of the monitor, and another EMG screen for continuous vagus nerve stimulation appears on the right side.

3. Standardization of intraoperative neuromonitoring

Adequate knowledge of the neuromonitoring system and standardization of the procedure are required for proper use of IONM [12–17]. In this context, both surgeons and anaesthesiologists are involved. In order to reach an adequate experience, it has been stated that the learning curve is approximately of 50–100 cases [18–20].

The anesthetist plays a key role in IONM procedure, particularly with regard to the type of drugs used to induce anaesthesia and to the positioning of the ET tube. After these steps, anesthesia can be obtained by inhaler or intravenous anesthetics: these agents do not have significant effects on EMG signal, providing an adequate depth of anesthesia. Differently, neuromuscular blocking agents (NMBAs) interfere with monitoring, reducing EMG amplitude and the optimal laryngeal response, thus making neuromonitoring less effective. For this reason, after induction, NMBA should be avoided for the rest of the operation. Small doses of a non-depolarizing muscle relaxant (usually rocuronium and atracurium) are used at intubation, as these agents allow the restoration of basic physiological functions, such as spontaneous respiration and normal muscle twitch activity, within a few minutes.

Endotracheal tubes are available in sizes 6.0, 6.5, 7.0, 7.5, and 8.0. The largest tube that can be passed between the patient's vocal cords has to be used. The ET tube is placed under direct laryngoscopy with the middle of the blue marked region (the exposed electrodes) in contact with the true vocal cords. The tube has to be placed in the right position to obtain adequate functioning of the system. Endotracheal tube positioning errors include not only depth errors but also rotational errors. The malposition of the ET can lead to misleading information and is a potential cause of loss of signal during surgery. After the tube is inserted, the patient is given the right operation position, with hyperextended neck, by applying a pillow under the shoulders. During positioning, the anesthetist must protect the ET tube to keep its position unchanged. If the tube is fixed to the rim of the patient's mouth before the patient is correctly positioned, the position of the tube in the airway can change. This can lead to a disruption of the relationship between the surface electrodes of the ET tube and the vocal cords. Thus, the tube has to be secured to the rim of the lip after the patient is correctly positioned.

Once the patient is positioned, the grounding electrode of the recording side and the grounding electrode of the stimulation side are subdermally applied to the presternal region or to the shoulder at the side of the monitor. The second one should be placed 1–2 cm below the first one.

After all connections are made, the correct positioning of the ET tube must be checked. This can be done from the monitor by verifying the impedance value of the electrodes (**Figure 4**). For each electrode, it has to be less than 5 kΩ. Moreover, the impedance difference between positive and negative electrodes of each channel should be less than 1 kΩ. Values above these thresholds indicate that the contact between the patient's vocal cords and the ET tube electrodes is not adequate. Other

DOI: http://dx.doi.org/10.5772/intechopen.83840

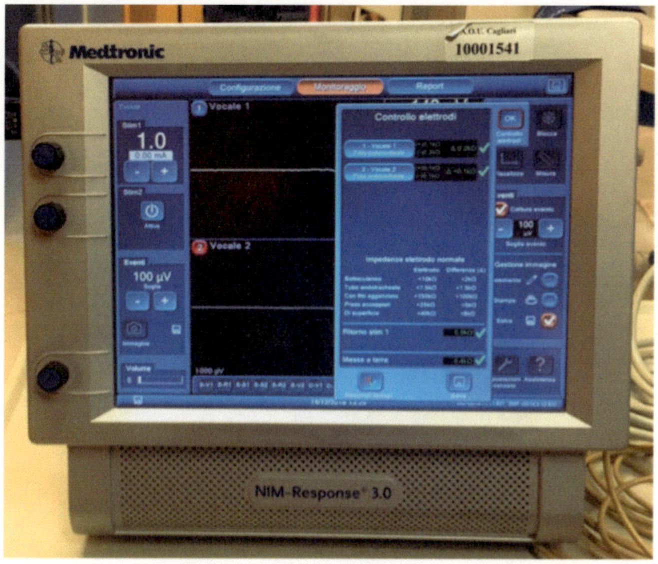

Figure 4.
Check of the impedance value of the electrodes from the monitor.

tests to verify the correct location of the ET tube include the evaluation of respiratory changes or a further laryngoscopy. About the first method, in the short-term window period between the loss of the effect of short-acting NMBA and the deepening of anesthesia following intubation, spontaneous respiratory movements should result in waveforms with an amplitude of 30–70 μV on the monitor. These respiratory changes should be detected for both vocal cords.

At this point, the monitor should be set as follows: a threshold value of 100 μV, an excitation electrode stimulation level of 0.5–2 mA (mean: 1 mA), a stimulation period of 100 μs, and a stimulation frequency of 4 stimuli per second.

At the beginning of the operation, the stimulator probe should be tested directly on the infrahyoid or sternocleidomastoid muscle to confirm the presence of an appropriate muscle twitching. This confirms that the nerve stimulation probe is working properly and the absence of ongoing paralytic agent. Moreover, to confirm the overall system function, before the identification of RLN, an EMG signal should initially be obtained from the vagus nerve. This step is crucial to assess that IONM system is functioning correctly and that the normal pathway of RLN signal is elicited. The vagus nerve can be directly stimulated after dissection of the carotid sheath, or its stimulation can be performed simply by increasing the stimulation level up to 2–3 mA with the probe on the carotid sheath without dissecting it. The RLN is situated at the tracheoesophageal groove in proximity to the inferior thyroid artery. It can be initially searched with a stimulation level of 2 mA and fully mapped out; then, it can be isolated and visually confirmed. Once the nerve is visualized, the stimulation level can be turned down to 1 mA. It is important to keep in mind that RLN extralaryngeal branching can be found in about 30–40% of patients, particularly at the level of Berry's ligament. Thus, it is necessary to dissect the RLN from the lower neck up to the nerve entrance into the larynx. In case of branched RLN, each branch should be stimulated separately by using a stimulation current of 0.4–0.5 mA. EMG signal of these individual branches should be assessed to allow a reliable evaluation of the distribution of the motor and sensory fibers. After removing the surgical specimen and ensuring a complete hemostasis, the final testing of RLN and vagus nerve is performed.

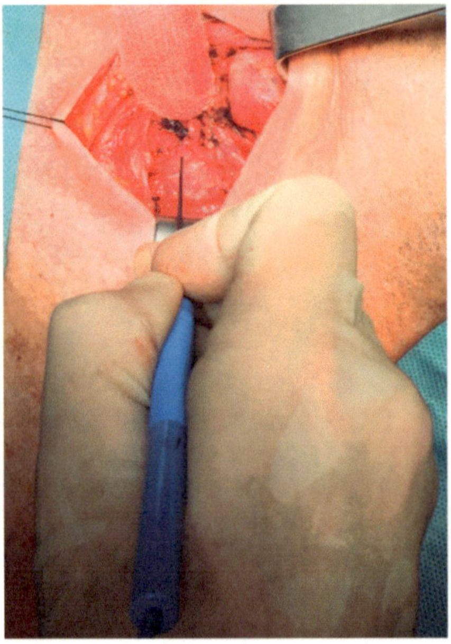

Figure 5.
RLN stimulation at the end of thyroid dissection and complete hemostasis (R2).

In 2011, the International Neural Monitoring Study Group (INMSG) defined the standard stages of intraoperative neuromonitoring in thyroid surgery by adding preoperative and postoperative vocal cord examinations to the four-step method previously proposed by Chiang et al. [12, 21]. The six stages can be summarized as follows:

a. preoperative laryngoscopy (L1);

b. vagus nerve stimulation before thyroidectomy (V1);

c. RLN stimulation upon initial identification (R1);

d. RLN stimulation at the end of thyroid dissection and complete hemostasis (R2) (**Figure** 5);

e. vagus nerve stimulation after complete thyroidectomy and hemostasis (V2);

f. postoperative laryngoscopy (L2).

As well as being useful during traditional open thyroidectomy, IONM can be very useful for RLN preservation also in case of endoscopic thyroid surgery [22, 23]. The fundamental steps of IONM during video-assisted thyroidectomy (VAT) are the same as those used during traditional thyroidectomy (L1, V1, R1, R2, V2, L2) [22]. IONM has proven to be very helpful also in the case of other endoscopic techniques, such as transaxillary or transoral thyroidectomy [23], even if a standardized technique is still lacking with these approaches.

4. Types of intraoperative neuromonitoring (I-IONM and C-IONM)

Currently, two types of IONM are available: the intermittent IONM (I-IONM) and the continuous IONM (C-IONM). With I-IONM, the functional integrity of the

RLN is limited to the site of direct nerve stimulation. For this reason, in proximal lesions of the RLN, distal stimulation near the larynx may produce a false negative IONM signal. Moreover, with this system, the RLN is at risk for damage during the time gap between two nerve stimulations. Ultimately, I-IONM allows the evaluation of the RLN only at the time of stimulation, and detects RLN lesion merely after it occurs [24].

To overcome these limits, a C-IONM technology has been introduced [25–28]. C-IONM consists in a probe that is applied directly to the vagus nerve, allowing the surgeon to constantly test the RLN function while dissecting the thyroid gland. However, the intermittent method is not a separate process from the continuous IONM technique. The intermittent IONM probe, in fact, is an integral and complementary part of the C-IONM [15]. The goal of continuous vagus nerve probing is to inform the surgeon immediately of any critical insult of the RLN, like traction, thus avoiding signal loss and vocal cord paralysis. A 50% decrease in amplitude and a 10% increase in latency time have been defined as critical changes [25, 28]. The device alarms when these thresholds are exceeded. According to recent observation, the most common cause of RLN lesion is tractional trauma [25–29]; C-IONM has proved to be useful in preventing traction injury by promptly detecting progressive decreases in EMG amplitude combined with progressive increases in latency. The surgeon can so avoid eventual RLN injury by changing his strategy. However, this system is not effective in case of acute injury of the nerve (section or thermal injury) [25–28].

5. Loss of signal

5.1 Definition of loss of signal

Loss of signal (LOS) occurs when the original EMG signal obtained from the vagus nerve and/or RLN nerve can no longer be elicited [12]. It is classified as true positive if vocal cord palsy is confirmed on postoperative laryngoscopy and false positive if no vocal cord palsy is present on postoperative laryngoscopy.

There are two types of LOS: the segmental type (Type 1) and the global type (Type 2).

Type 1 LOS consists in the loss of signal at a certain point in the nerve; signal is obtained distally to the point where the nerve is injured, but no signal is detected proximally to this site.

In case of Type 2 LOS, instead, no specific damage point is recognizable, and no signal is acquired stimulating the RLN all along its course or stimulating the vagus nerve.

About this argument, it is important to introduce another concept: the intraoperative signal recovery. Especially with the introduction of the C-IONM with continuous vagus nerve stimulation, it has been noted that, in some patients with signal loss, the signal can improve in the course of the operation.

5.2 Troubleshooting algorithm for loss of signal

When LOS occurs, a troubleshooting protocol should be followed to check the IONM system for technical problems [13, 30, 31].

In this case, the first procedure to be performed is to palpate the larynx with a finger behind the posterior plate of the cricoid to feel the posterior cricoarytenoid muscle contraction in response to RLN stimulation.

If digital detection of the laryngeal twitch is present in response to nerve stimulation, the stimulation side of the system is working properly, and a malfunction of the recording side should be considered. The most frequent causes of malfunction of the recording side are ET tube malposition, displacement of grounding electrodes, or malfunction of the ET tube electrodes.

In addition to laryngeal palpation, contralateral vagal assessment also represents a useful option for troubleshooting. If contralateral vagus nerve stimulation does not elicit an adequate EMG signal, a malfunction of the recording side should be investigated as first option. Differently, if the contralateral vagus nerve is properly functioning, a possible nerve lesion must be considered.

If laryngeal twitch is absent when the nerve is stimulated, a malfunction of the stimulation side should be considered, thus the nerve stimulator probe and monitor have to be checked. Nerve stimulator probe function should be checked by applying its tip directly on a muscle to confirm a muscle twitching. Moreover, the whole system, with special attention focused on the monitor screen, must be fully reviewed. Again, with regard to stimulation side error, if C-IONM is used, LOS may be due to a dislocation of the vagal nerve electrode.

Finally, in case of LOS, it is of fundamental importance to rule any administration of NMBA during the operation.

6. Advantages and limits of IONM

6.1 Advantages of IONM

Visualization of RLNs is considered the gold standard in thyroid surgery to reduce the incidence of nerve palsy. Nevertheless, visualization of the nerve can only suggest an anatomic integrity, which does not ensure functionality. In fact, some studies have demonstrated that the most common mechanism of nerve injury is traction [29, 32], resulting in a palsy with complete anatomic integrity. Furthermore, direct visualization of the nerve can be difficult, especially in case of revision neck surgery, because of the scar tissue [1, 32–34], in case of anatomic variations of the nerve, during central compartment lymph node dissection, or in course of surgery for advanced thyroid cancer. For these reasons, in the last decades, the use of IONM has widely spread among endocrine surgeons, in order to facilitate identification and dissection of the nerve and to evaluate its functionality, predicting vocal cord function outcome.

However, to date, studies have failed to demonstrate a statistically significant reduction of incidence of nerve injury using IONM [2, 3]; this lack of data may be related to the very low rate of nerve palsy. It has been estimated that in prospective, randomized trials, the calculated sample size needed to demonstrate that incidence of palsy is lower with IONM use is about 9000 nerves at risk [1, 7]. Other authors have reported that at least 39,000 nerves at risk per arm should be necessary to achieve statistical power that could demonstrate a significant difference in RLN palsy rate [3]. To date, only one randomized controlled trial [35] has demonstrated a significant reduction of transient RLN palsy from 5 to 2.7% ($p = 0.007$).

Furthermore, it is important to underline that voice impairment isn't always due to RLN palsy; other causes can be vocal cord damage due to orotracheal intubation and damage of the strap muscles. In these cases, the good surgical practice and the integrity and functionality of the nerve are assessed by IONM, preserving from medical claim.

Advantages of IONM of RLNs in thyroid surgery are:

- Early identification of RLN and aid in dissection: Stimulation of paratracheal area allows to identify the course of the nerve before it is visualized; the identified area is then carefully dissected until the nerve is satisfactorily exposed.

Once the nerve is identified, stimulation of the adjacent structures can help to distinguish the nerve from other non-neural elements, like vessels. IONM is also helpful in identifying neural branches and to clarify nerve course in case of anatomic variants.

- Intraoperative diagnosis of RLN injury and postoperative prognosis: The most common causes of RLN injuries are transection of the nerve, suture entrapment, traction, compression, contusion, pressure, ischemia by excessive skeletization, thermal trauma caused by dissection or hemostatic instruments used too close to the nerve. In most of the cases of nerve injury, the nerve is anatomically intact, thus visualization only is not predictive of a vocal cord palsy; on the contrary, IONM allows to predict most of the nerve injuries, improving the accuracy of prognostic evaluation of nerve functionality. Once a loss of signal is detected, IONM allows to identify with high accuracy the site of the lesion by stimulating the nerve all long its course and the vagus nerve.

- Reduction of bilateral RLN palsy: Once RLN palsy has been diagnosed with IONM on the first side of resection, the surgeon can decide to modify the initially scheduled bilateral surgery and to perform a delayed completion thyroidectomy (two-staged thyroidectomy), in order to avoid a bilateral RLN palsy.

- Difficult cases: IONM has beneficial effects especially in difficult cases, like reoperative surgery, locally advanced thyroid cancer and cervico-mediastinal goiter, or in case of lymphadenectomy of central neck compartment, facilitating identification and dissection of the nerve.

- Improvement of radicality in total thyroidectomy: Most of RLN injuries are produced during dissection of thyroid tissue from Berry ligament, within the last 2 cm of the nerve. The two main reasons of lesion are a ramification of RLN, which occurs usually less than 5 mm of its entry in larynx, or an intracapsular course of RLN, which is reported in 15–38% of cases. Thus, in the absence of IONM, surgeons often tend to leave a small amount of thyroid tissue to avoid lesion of RLN in the last part of its course. On the contrary, IONM allows to completely resect the thyroid gland, reducing the risk of nerve palsy. Furthermore, hemostatic maneuvers can be safely conducted with IONM, ensuring that surgical sutures do not exert a traction on the nerve and that cauterization is far enough from the nerve.

6.2 Limits of IONM

The first evidence is that, despite IONM usage, RLN injury still remains one of the most common complications in thyroid surgery. Multiple studies have failed to demonstrate a reduction of incidence of RLN injury when IONM is used in thyroid surgery; as already discussed, this may be due to the very low incidence of RLN palsy. Surgeon should be conscious that IONM does not prevent at all RLN injury. In fact, stimulation of the nerve can assure integrity of the nerve only after dissection, while nerve palsy can be identified only after the injury has been produced. Thus, IONM should be considered an adjunct, but direct visualization of the nerve and careful dissection of the tissues are needed.

Although the specificity of IONM in detecting nerve injury is very high (94–99%), a small number of patients will have a vocal cord dysfunction despite regular neuromonitoring signal (false-negative IONM). By the other side, a loss of signal (LOS) at the end of procedure is predictive of a postoperative vocal cord paralysis, but positive predictive value ranges widely from 33 to 90%.; this is probably related to the poor uniformity in application of IONM across different centers. It has been reported that preoperative and postoperative laryngoscopy is performed routinely only in 15% of centers who use IONM [36], and that vagal stimulation is not routinely performed in most of the centers [37]. Furthermore, usage of IONM needs a learning curve, a precise knowledge of the components and of the issues that may occur: insufficient experience in managing IONM may result in misleading information that can increase the risk of RLN injury.

The most frequent causes of false negative results are malposition of endotracheal tube, technical problems related to stimulation or registration devices, neuromuscular blocking due to anaesthetic drugs; another cause of false positive result is thought to be transient neuropraxia with rapid recovery before end of surgery.

Thus, low positive predictive value is the main limit of IONM. A low positive predictive value means that, in the worst-case scenario, two out of three patients with LOS will not suffer any alteration of vocal cord motility after surgery. In this regard, a standardization of IONM methods and reporting has been undertaken to provide uniformity and to minimize variations in application of IONM. As already discussed, standardization of IONM should include pre- and postoperative laryngoscopy, stimulation of vagus nerve before dissection and at the end of surgery, and stimulation of RLN when identified and at the end of lobectomy.

7. Two-staged thyroidectomy

Routine use of IONM in thyroid surgery has led to two-stage operations to prevent bilateral RLN palsy. This approach is defined as removal of the thyroid gland in two different procedures: in the first one, surgery is limited to the main lobe, while the remnant gland is excised in a second intervention. In fact, in case of LOS after excision of the first lobe, the surgeon can evaluate the opportunity to delay removal of the second lobe. Thus, a LOS during first lobectomy should induce to consider timing for contralateral lobectomy. This decision should take into account several elements, including especially thyroid pathology. Over the years, oncologic radicality in case of two-staged thyroidectomy has been a matter of debate; in this regard, we should consider that differentiated thyroid tumors have a good prognosis even in case of local or distant metastases, and that radioablative therapy with iodine-131 can be delayed safely. Thus two-staged thyroidectomy seems to be adequate also in case of thyroid carcinoma [38]; in this case, the endocrinologist can prescribe a TSH-suppressive therapy to reduce the risk of tumor progression of eventually unresected foci of tumor. Alternatively, a near-total lobectomy could be performed on the second side to preserve contralateral RLN. In this scenario, it is necessary to underline once again the importance of a correct standardization of IONM to reduce false positive results; that may lead to an unnecessary two-staged thyroidectomy. In case of thyroid cancer, thyroidectomy should always begin from tumoral side, or, in case of bilateral carcinoma, from the side where the nodule has more aggressive features. In case of two-staged thyroidectomy, contralateral lobectomy should be carefully planned after recovery of vocal cord motility, typically 6–8 weeks after surgery, or, in case of permanent palsy, after demonstration of enough respiratory space.

8. Conclusions

IONM is a valuable instrument in thyroid surgery. A correct standardization of the method is necessary to reduce the number of false positive results. In case of loss of signal, two-staged thyroidectomy can be safely performed even in case of malignancy.

Conflict of interest

The authors declare that there is no conflict of interest.

Author details

Fabio Medas*, Gian Luigi Canu, Enrico Erdas and Pietro Giorgio
Department of Surgical Sciences, University of Cagliari, Italy

*Address all correspondence to: fabiomedas@gmail.com

IntechOpen

© 2019 The Author(s). Licensee IntechOpen. This chapter is distributed under the terms of the Creative Commons Attribution License (http://creativecommons.org/licenses/by/3.0), which permits unrestricted use, distribution, and reproduction in any medium, provided the original work is properly cited.

References

[1] Deniwar A, Kandil E, Randolph G. Electrophysiological neural monitoring of the laryngeal nerves in thyroid surgery: Review of the current literature. Gland Surgery. 2015;**4**:368-375. DOI: 10.3978/j.issn.2227-684X.2015.04.04

[2] Pisanu A, Porceddu G, Podda M, Cois A, Uccheddu A. Systematic review with metaanalysis of studies comparing intraoperative neuromonitoring of recurrent laryngeal nerves versus visualization alone during thyroidectomy. The Journal of Surgical Research. 2014;**188**:152-161. DOI: 10.1016/j.jss.2013.12.022

[3] Deniwar A, Bhatia P, Kandil E. Electrophysiological neuromonitoring of the laryngeal nerves in thyroid and parathyroid surgery: A review. World Journal of Experimental Medicine. 2015;**5**:120-123. DOI: 10.5493/wjem.v5.i2.120

[4] Gurrado A, Bellantone R, Cavallaro G, Citton M, Constantinides V, Conzo G, et al. Can total thyroidectomy be safely performed by residents?: A comparative retrospective multicenter study. Medicine (Baltimore). 2016;**95**:e3241. DOI: 10.1097/MD.0000000000003241

[5] Goretzki PE, Schwarz K, Brinkmann J, Wirowski D, Lammers BJ. The impact of intraoperative neuromonitoring (IONM) on surgical strategy in bilateral thyroid diseases: Is it worth the effort? World Journal of Surgery. 2010;**34**: 1274-1284. DOI: 10.1007/s00268-009-0353-3

[6] Jeannon JP, Orabi AA, Bruch GA, Abdalsalm HA, Simo R. Diagnosis of recurrent laryngeal nerve palsy after thyroidectomy: A systematic review. International Journal of Clinical Practice. 2009;**63**:624-629. DOI: 10.1111/j.1742-1241.2008.01875.x

[7] Dralle H, Lorenz K, Machens A. Verdicts on malpractice claims after thyroid surgery: Emerging trends and future directions. Head & Neck. 2012;**34**:1591-1596. DOI: 10.1002/hed.21970

[8] Rosato L, Avenia N, Bernante P, De Palma M, Gulino G, Nasi PG, et al. Complications of thyroid surgery: Analysis of a multicentric study on 14,934 patients operated on in Italy over 5 years. World Journal of Surgery. 2004;**28**:271-276. DOI: 10.1007/s00268-003-6903-1

[9] Bergenfelz A, Jansson S, Kristoffersson A, Mårtensson H, Reihnér E, Wallin G, et al. Complications to thyroid surgery: Results as reported in a database from a multicentre audit comprising 3660 patients. Langenbeck's Archives of Surgery. 2008;**393**:667-673. DOI: 10.1007/s00423-008-0366-7

[10] Snyder SK, Lairmore TC, Hendricks JC, Roberts JW. Elucidating mechanisms of recurrent laryngeal nerve injury during thyroidectomy and parathyroidectomy. Journal of the American College of Surgeons. 2008;**206**:123130. DOI: 10.1016/j.jamcollsurg.2007.07.017

[11] Melin M, Schwarz K, Pearson MD, Lammers BJ, Goretzki PE. Postoperative vocal cord dysfunction despite normal intraoeprative neuromonitoring: An unexpected complication with the risk of bilateral palsy. World Journal of Surgery. 2014;**38**:2597-2602. DOI: 10.1007/s00268-014-2591-2

[12] Randolph GW, Dralle H, International Intraoperative Monitoring Study Group, Abdullah H, Barczynski M, Bellantone R, et al. Electrophysiologic recurrent laryngeal nerve monitoring during thyroid and parathyroid surgery: International

standards guideline statement. The Laryngoscope. 2011;**121**(S1):Suppl 1-Suppl16. DOI: 10.1002/lary.21119

[13] Durán Poveda M, Dionigi G, Sitges-Serra A, Barczynski M, Angelos P, Dralle H, et al. Intraoperative monitoring of the recurrent laryngeal nerve during thyroidectomy: A standardized approach part 2. World Journal of Endocrine Surgery. 2012;**4**:33-40. DOI: 10.5005/jp-journals-10002-1091

[14] Uludag M, Aygun N, Kaya C, Tanal M, Oba S, Isgor A. Basic principles and standardization of intraoperative nerve monitoring in thyroid surgery. The Medical Bulletin of Sisli Etfal Hospital. 2017;**51**:13-25. DOI: 10.5350/SEMB.20170216084444

[15] Dionigi G, Wu CW, Lombardi D, Accorona R, Bozzola A, Kim HY, et al. The current state of recurrent laryngeal nerve monitoring for thyroid surgery. Current Otorhinolaryngology Reports. 2014;**2**:44-54. DOI: 10.1007/s40136-013-0033-6

[16] Shedd DP, Durham C. Electrical identification of the recurrent laryngeal nerve. I. Response of the canine larynx to electrical stimulation of the recurrent laryngeal nerve. Annals of Surgery. 1966;**163**:47-50

[17] Calò PG, Medas F, Gordini L, Podda F, Erdas E, Pisano G, et al. Interpretation of intraoperative recurrent laryngeal nerve monitoring signals: The importance of a correct standardization. International Journal of Surgery. 2016;**28**(Suppl 1):S54-S58. DOI:10.1016/j.ijsu.2015.12.039

[18] Dionigi G, Bacuzzi A, Boni L, Rovera F, Dionigi R. What is the learning curve for intraoperative neuromonitoring in thyroid surgery? International Journal of Surgery. 2008;**6**(Suppl 1):S7-S12. DOI: 10.1016/j.ijsu.2008.12.023

[19] Jonas J, Bähr R. Intraoperative neuromonitoring of the recurrent laryngeal nerve—Results and learning curve. Zentralblatt für Chirurgie. 2006;**131**:443-448. DOI: 10.1055/s-2006-955453

[20] Pragacz K, Barczyński M. Evaluation of the learning curve for intraoperative neural monitoring of the recurrent laryngeal nerves in thyroid surgery. Polski Przeglad Chirurgiczny. 2015;**86**:584-593. DOI: 10.1515/pjs-2015-0005

[21] Chiang FY, Lee KW, Chen HC, Chen HY, Lu IC, Kuo WR, et al. Standardization of intraoperative neuromonitoring of recurrent laryngeal nerve in thyroid operation. World Journal of Surgery. 2010;**34**:223-229. DOI: 10.1007/s00268-009-0316-8

[22] Dionigi G, Boni L, Rovera F, Bacuzzi A, Dionigi R. Neuromonitoring and video-assisted thyroidectomy: A prospective, randomized case-control evaluation. Surgical Endoscopy. 2009;**23**:996-1003. DOI: 10.1007/s00464-008-0098-3

[23] Lang BH, Wong KP. Feasibility on the use of intraoperative vagal nerve stimulation in gasless, transaxillary endoscopic, and robotic-assisted thyroidectomy. Journal of Laparoendoscopic & Advanced Surgical Techniques. Part A. 2011;**21**:911-917. DOI: 10.1089/lap.2011.0204

[24] Dionigi G, Van Slycke S, Boni L, Rausei S, Mangano A. Limits of neuromonitoring in thyroid surgery. Annals of Surgery. 2013;**258**:e1-e2. DOI: 10.1097/SLA.0b013e318294559d

[25] Schneider R, Przybyl J, Pliquett U, Hermann M, Wehner M, Pietsch UC, et al. A new vagal anchor electrode for real-time monitoring of the recurrent laryngeal nerve. American Journal of Surgery. 2010;**199**:507514. DOI: 10.1016/j.amjsurg.2009.04.036

[26] Schneider R, Bures C, Lorenz K, Dralle H, Freissmuth M, Hermann M. Evolution of nerve injury with unexpected EMG signal recovery in thyroid surgery using continuous intraoperative neuromonitoring. World Journal of Surgery. 2013;**37**:364-368. DOI: 10.1007/s00268-012-1853-0

[27] Lamadé W, Ulmer C, Friedrich C, Rieber F, Schymik K, Gemkow HM, et al. Signal stability as key requirement for continuous intraoperative neuromonitoring. Der Chirurg. 2011;**82**:913-920. DOI: 10.1007/s00104-011-2080-1

[28] Schneider R, Randolph GW, Sekulla C, Phelan E, Thanh PN, Bucher M, et al. Continuous intraoperative vagus nerve stimulation for identification of imminent recurrent laryngeal nerve injury. Head & Neck. 2013;**35**:1591-1598. DOI: 10.1002/hed.23187

[29] Dionigi G, Wu CW, Kim HY, Rausei S, Boni L, Chiang FY. Severity of recurrent laryngeal nerve injuries in thyroid surgery. World Journal of Surgery. 2016;**40**:1373-1381. DOI: 10.1007/s00268-016-3415-3

[30] Randolph GW, Kobler JB, Wilkins J. Recurrent laryngeal nerve identification and assessment during thyroid surgery: Laryngeal palpation. World Journal of Surgery. 2004;**28**:755-760. DOI: 10.1007/s00268-004-7348-x

[31] Tomoda C, Hirokawa Y, Uruno T, Takamura Y, Ito Y, Miya A, et al. Sensitivity and specificity of intraoperative recurrent laryngeal nerve stimulation test for predicting vocal cord palsy after thyroid surgery. World Journal of Surgery. 2006;**30**:1230-1233. DOI: 10.1007/s00268-005-0351-z

[32] Calò PG, Pisano G, Medas F, Marcialis J, Gordini L, Erdas E, et al. Total thyroidectomy without prophylactic central neck dissection in clinically node-negative papillary thyroid cancer: Is it an adequate treatment? World Journal of Surgical Oncology. 2014;**12**:152. DOI: 10.1186/1477-7819-12-152

[33] Calò PG, Pisano G, Medas F, Tatti A, Tuveri M, Nicolosi A. Risk factors in reoperative thyroid surgery for recurrent goiter: Our experience. Il Giornale di Chirurgia. 2012;**33**:335-338

[34] Pironi D, Pontone S, Vendettuoli M, Podzemny V, Mascagni D, Arcieri S, et al. Prevention of complications during reoperative thyroid surgery. La Clinica Terapeutica. 2014;**165**:e285-e290. DOI: 10.7417/CT.2014.1744

[35] Barczynski M, Konturek A, Cichon S. Randomized clinical trial of visualization versus neuromonitoring of recurrent laryngeal nerves during thyroidectomy. The British Journal of Surgery. 2009;**96**:240-246. DOI: 10.1002/bjs.6417

[36] Dionigi G, Tanda ML, Piantanida E, Boni L, Rovera F, Dionigi R, et al. Time interval in diagnosis and treatment of papillary thyroid cancer: A descriptive, retrospective study. American Journal of Surgery. 2009;**197**:434-438. DOI: 10.1016/j.amjsurg.2008.01.031

[37] Dionigi G, Bacuzzi A, Barczynski M, Biondi A, Boni L, Chiang FY, et al. Implementation of systematic neuromonitoring training for thyroid surgery. Updates in Surgery. 2011;**63**:201-207. DOI: 10.1007/s13304-011-0098-z

[38] Calò PG, Medas F, Conzo G, Podda F, Canu GL, Gambardella C, et al. Intraoperative neuromonitoring in thyroid surgery: Is the two-staged thyroidectomy justified? International Journal of Surgery. 2017;**41**(Suppl 1):S13-S20. DOI: 10.1016/j.ijsu.2017.02.001

Chapter 7

Genetic Alterations of RET: Possible Implications and Clinical Correlations in Thyroid Carcinogenesis

Syed Mudassar, Mosin S. Khan, Shariq R. Masoodi, Mahboob Ul Hussain and Khurshid I. Andrabi

Abstract

Thyroid cancers are malignant tumors in the thyroid gland. DNA polymorphisms are playing a decisive role in unscrambling the genomic basis of tumor formation and development in cancer. Thyroid cancer is influenced in a polygenic and low-penetrance manner by *RET* gene polymorphisms and this part of the world (North India) has not recorded any study regarding *RET* alterations in this very cancer. We assessed *RET* G691S (*rs*1799939), L769L (*rs*1800861) and S904S (*rs*1800863) polymorphisms by restriction fragment length polymorphism (RFLP) in order to explain their potential role in the diagnosis and prognosis of Papillary thyroid cancer (PTC) and follicular thyroid cancer (FTC). In RET G691S polymorphism, the total dissemination of variant alleles (GA + AA) was 62.9% in cases as related to 44.5% in controls ($P < 0.05$). *RET* L769L variant alleles (TG + GG) was 70% in cases versus 88% in controls ($P < 0.05$). In *RET* S904S, occurrence of variant alleles (CG + GG) was 56% in cases versus 44% in controls ($P < 0.05$). G691S and L769L polymorphism advocate a "Dominant mode of inheritance". The S904S polymorphism approves an "Additive mode of inheritance". In conclusion, there was an over-representation of *RET* G691S/S904S polymorphisms and under-representation of L769L polymorphism in PTC and FTC patients. Additionally, our data suggest that some haplotypes (A T G, G T G and A T C) of *RET* may act as low penetrance alleles for predisposition of thyroid cancer.

Keywords: thyroid cancer, rearranged during transfection, RET, polymorphism, papillary thyroid cancer, follicular thyroid cancer

1. Introduction

Cancer is a large group of diseases that vary in their age of onset, rate of growth, state of cellular differentiation, diagnostic detectability, invasiveness, metastatic potential, response to treatment, and prognosis. However, cancer may be a relatively small number of diseases caused by similar molecular defects in cell function resulting from common types of alterations to a cell's genes as per molecular and cell biological point of view. Ultimately, abnormal gene expression causes cancer which may occur due to mutation, translocation, amplification, deletion, loss of heterozygosity, etc. Cell replication and cell death in a tumor cell population gets imbalanced leading to an expansion of tumor tissue [1, 2].

The most common malignancy of the endocrine system is Thyroid cancer. 2% of all diagnosed cancer cases and majority of endocrine cancer related deaths each year are due to this cancer type [3–5].

The rearranged during transfection (*RET*) proto-oncogene expressed in cells of neural crest origin and encodes a membrane tyrosine-kinase receptor [6]. However, thyroid follicular cells may also express the *RET* tyrosine kinase domain [7]. Somatic *RET* translocations were found in some sporadic and radiation-induced PTCs. Papillary thyroid cancer contains *RET/PTC* chromosomal rearrangement [8]. In this gene rearrangement, a portion of the *RET* gene is fused to one of several genes. *RET/PTC1* and *RET/PTC3* are the most common rearrangement types in which *RET* is fused to *CCDC6* (also known as *H4*) or *NCOA4* (also known as *ELE1* or *RFG*) respectively [9, 10]. *RET* tyrosine kinase domain gets constitutively activated due to *RET* rearrangement that can lead to PTC [11, 12]. 10–20% of sporadic PTC's contain RET/PTC rearrangements. Patients with the history of radiation exposure (50–80%), PTC's from children and young adults (40–70%) have higher frequency of *RET/PTC* rearrangements [13, 14].

Genetic basis of tumor formation and cancer progression is being unraveled by DNA polymorphisms. The human genome as a whole (in which over 3.1 million sequence variations have been mapped), represent 25–35% of the total estimated SNPs [15]. Predisposition to several human cancers is due to polymorphisms. Apart from *RET* rearrangements, the coding sequence of *RET* display polymorphisms in exon 2 (G135A, A45A), in exon 7 (G1296A, A432A), in exon 11 (G2071A, G691S), in exon 13 (T2307G, L769L), in exon 14 (C2508T, S836S), and in exon 15 (C2712G, S904S) [16, 17]. Etiology of sporadic Hirschsprung disease (HSCR) and MTC has been associated with *RET* polymorphisms [18–20]. Silent *RET* polymorphisms; A45A in exon 2 and L769L in exon 13 may represent low-penetrance risk in PTC [20]. Risk of differentiated thyroid cancer with reference to *RET* Polymorphic Haplotypes was also reported by some studies [21]. The mechanisms by which the silent polymorphisms may act in the development of cancer include transcript stability, RNA splicing, and DNA protein binding and protein folding.

The valley of Kashmir is one of the divisions of Jammu and Kashmir State, situated in the Himalayas. Kashmir, regarded worldwide as paradise on earth, with over 07 million populations is heavily burdened with different organ cancers. In Kashmir valley where incidences of almost all types of organ cancers have shown a drastic increase in last couple of decades particularly GIT and lung cancers, the thyroid cancer figures no less in this deadly race. Thyroid cancer is the 8th most common cancer and 7th most common cancer among women in Kashmir valley. The frequency of thyroid cancer has increased from 2.3% in 1995 to 5.4% in 2010 in Kashmir valley [22]. Also, owing to the fact that there is no data on genetic alterations in thyroid cancer available in our population and given the backdrop of a significant presence of thyroid cancer patients, it is the first initiative to study the gene alterations in Thyroid cancer patients of Kashmir Valley. In view of these observations this study was designed to address the disease pathology associated with the thyroid cancer through the Polymorphic analysis of RET gene SNPs—G691S (G2071A), L769L (T2307G) and S904S (C2712G) in order to observe pattern of association of various SNPs G691S (G2071A), L769L (T2307G) and S904S (C2712G) of RET gene in thyroid cancer.

2. DNA polymorphisms in thyroid cancer

The ability to visualize sequence differences directly in DNA is one of the most important tools underlying the revolution in medical genetics. Polymorphisms are these differences in DNA sequences when studied in the context of a population which may be present in exons (coding regions) or introns (noncoding) regions of genes. Family studies have been undergone by studying the genes of medical importance through visualizing thousands of DNA polymorphisms.

Characteristically, polymorphisms denote sequence variations which confer no deleterious effects and are present in the general population. However, as molecular epidemiological studies were performed and the human genome project was deciphered it became vibrant that some "polymorphisms" were not entirely harmless. Genes for many disorders with a clear pattern of Mendelian inheritance were located and identified by this technique, such as, muscular dystrophies, cystic fibrosis and neurodegenerative disorders and This technique also assists in finding genes that predispose people to diseases in which inheritance patterns are complex, such as diabetes, atherosclerosis, and hypertension. These polymorphisms are crucial in the identification of genes important for susceptibility to common cancers, such as colon cancer, as well as susceptibility to less common childhood tumors, such as retinoblastoma and Wilms' tumor [23]. Over 3.1 million sequence variations have been mapped in the human genome in which, 25–35% of the total estimated SNPs are present [15, 24]. Individual susceptibility is likely due to genetic factors modulating the environmental risk otherwise differentiated thyroid cancer is described by a strong hereditability, hence, the identification of genetic variations is important for understanding the possible mechanisms tangled in thyroid carcinogenesis. In thyroid cancer many single nucleotide polymorphisms have been reported in different genes and functional analysis of many single nucleotide polymorphisms have been carried out. It has been reported that these DNA polymorphisms in various genes predispose a person to higher risk of thyroid cancer and also has a marked effect on various clinicopathological characteristics of thyroid cancer patients [23].

3. Structure and biology of RET receptor

Located on chromosome 10q11.2 near the centromere, the *RET* gene includes 21 exons. *RET* (rearranged during transfection) was first identified by Takahashi et al. in 1985 as a proto-oncogene that can undergo activation by cytogenic rearrangement [25]. *RET* gene was cloned by the same investigators 3 years later [26]. This gene encodes the RET receptor, a plasma membrane-bound tyrosine kinase enzyme. RET gene is expressed by neuroendocrine and neural cells, including parasympathetic, sympathetic and colonic ganglia, cells of the urogenital tract, thyroid C cells, adrenal medullary cells and parathyroid cells derived from branchial arches [27, 28]. The RET protein contains two intracellular tyrosine kinase domains, a transmembrane domain, an extracellular region (four cadherin-like repeats, a calcium binding site, and a cysteine-rich domain) and N terminal signal peptide. The cysteine-rich extracellular domain is central for receptor dimerization, whereas, the extracellular cadherin-like domains are key for cell-cell signaling. The RET C-terminal tail shows three splicing variants producing three protein isoforms with 9 (RET9; short isoform), 43 (RET43; middle isoform), or 51 (RET51; long

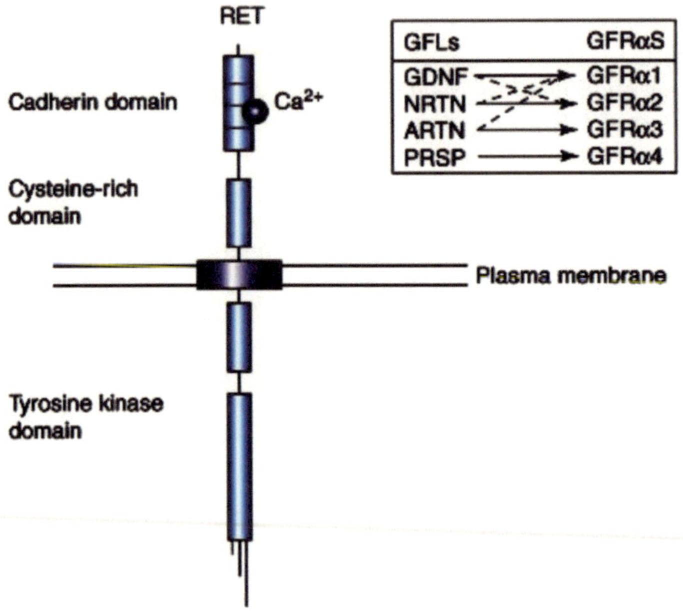

Figure 1.
The RET protein, its functional domains, ligands and co-receptors. Left, *functional domains of the three RET isoforms.* Right, *canonical (unbroken lines) and noncanonical (broken lines) interactions of the RET ligands GDNF, neurturin (NRTN), persephin (PSPN) and artemin (ARTN) with their GFRa co-receptors. Lipid rafts are depicted as a purple box in the plasma membrane.*

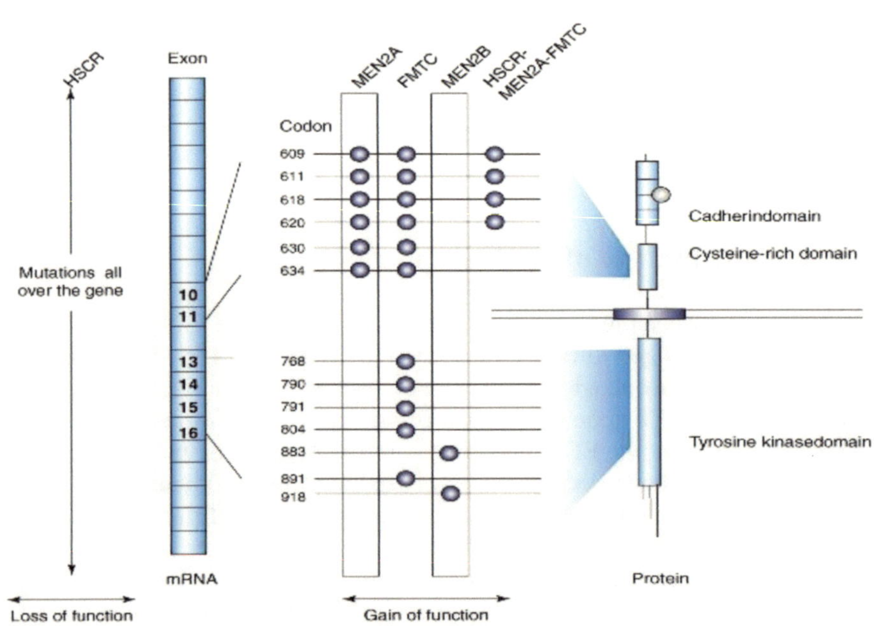

Figure 2.
Germline missense mutations in RET associated with MEN2 and Hirschsprung disease (HSCR). Shown are the structure of the RET mRNA and protein. The codons mutated, the associated clinical entities, and the location of these mutations in relation to the exons and structural domains are indicated.

isoform) distinct amino acids at their C termini [29, 30] (**Figure 1**). Four ligands for the *RET* receptor have been recognized so far [31, 32]. These ligands are *persephin*, *artemin*, *neurturin* and the *glial cell line-derived neurotrophic factor* (*GDNF*) [33, 34]. **Figure 2** summarizes various *RET* mutations along with disease phenotype.

4. Polymorphisms and haplotypes in RET

RET polymorphisms are might be associated with an increased relative risk for the development of disorders derived from neural crest cells and are believed to be genetic modifiers. High penetrant germline *RET* mutations have a key role in disease development. Various disease phenotypes have relatively strong association with *RET* polymorphisms. The most common *RET* polymorphisms; the nonsynonymous variant in exon 11 (G691S; G2071A) and the synonymous variants in exon 13 (L767L; T2307G), in exon 14 (S836S; C2508T) and in exon 15 (S904S; C2712G), are being denoted as disease modifiers due to their presence in patients with sporadic MTC and DTC [35–37]. Disease-associated germline mutations might interact with these polymorphisms or other genetic variants, tempering the age of onset or disease phenotype. Polymorphisms could bestow a much higher attributable risk on the general population as compared with rare mutations in high-penetrance *RET* gene. G691S and S904S polymorphisms of *RET* have a transformer effect on the age of onset of MEN2A [38]. Sporadic MTC has been associated with several *RET* polymorphisms [39]. A low-penetrance *RET* haplotype comprising the wild-type allele at IVS1-126 and IVS1-1463 and a 16-basepair intron-1 deletion of these SNPs is strongly associated with and over represented in *sporadic pheochromocytoma* [40]. *Hirschsprung disease* has disease associated polymorphisms linked to it [41, 42]. Two closely located SNPs, rs2435357 and rs2506004, in intron 1 has been observed by two groups as disease-causing candidates on the basis of comparative genomics, functional assays and association studies [43, 44]. G691S and S904S linkage have been proposed previously [45]. G691S/S904S cosegregated together as haplotype ($P < 0.001$) in one of the studies, proposing that these polymorphisms are in linkage disequilibrium with each other [46].

5. RET polymorphisms and haplotypes in differentiated thyroid cancers

Follicular and parafollicular-type C cells were shown to have some interconnections. The MTC cells provide the microenvironment that has the capacity to stimulate the proliferation of follicular cells, resulting in hyperplastic and adenomatous follicles which could ultimately acquire a fully developed neoplastic phenotype. Some patients with Hashimoto thyroiditis had C-cell hyperplasia [47, 48]. *RET* receptor has been shown to express in thyroid follicular component, which may be activated in the existence of precise ligands in the thyroid microenvironment.

Presence of RET ligands in this microenvironment is highly reasonable because C cells express the RET receptor. Follicular cell derived thyroid cancers contain *RET* mRNA which may be activated in the presence of specific ligands [7]. So the role of *RET* gene polymorphism in differentiated thyroid cancers came into existence. Some variants within *RET* could represent low penetrant alleles for the PTC phenotype. A study revealed the toughest association of A45A (G135A) and L769L (T2307G) with PTC [20]. Borrego et al. described the seven most frequent haplotypes in cases and controls and some of which differed in their distribution [19]. The G G C C haplotype is over-represented in both populations of sporadic PTC.

G allele of exon 2 and the G allele of exon 13 are included in the G G C C haplotype. A432A and S836S polymorphisms had strongest association with DTC as per the study conducted by Lesueur et al. Yet, the scale of the detected effect between DTC and *RET* SNPs was modest [20].

The mechanism by which these silent polymorphisms act and develop *RET* related diseases is still a question of debate. *First*, stability of protein synthesis could be disturbed by such genetic sequence variations through influence on RNA splicing, hence, a new cryptic splice acceptor, donor, or enhancer site could be formed which could result in a receptor that did not bind ligand well or in a truncated protein [49]. *RET* A45A polymorphism may result in alternative splicing and produce a mRNA isoforms as per Borrego et al. [49]. They further hypothesized that decreased protein expression on the cell surface could be due to these RNA isoforms, erroneous ligand binding, microRNA binding, change of structure/copies and mRNA stability synthesis of incomplete proteins and also the change in the structure of proteins caused by slowing down of translation [50, 51]. However, homozygosity confers the phenotypically evident changes [49]. *Second*, other nearby mutations could be influenced by these silent polymorphisms. *Third*, the polymorphism may incline to decreased expression of the variant allele, thus leading to low level functional haplo insufficiency. *Fourth*, these polymorphisms may lie in linkage disequilibrium with other sequences that may directly confer low level predisposition to or protection against disease. *Fifth*, slightly decreased efficiency of RET translation may be due to preferential usage of tRNA molecules. The variant(s) is less favored and the wild type would be the favored sequence. *Sixth*, *RET* gene will be susceptible to damage by environmental insults such as radiation by these silent polymorphisms [21]. *Finally*, mRNA conservation in the case of presence of various polymorphic variants in the *RET* gene based on bioinformatics methods is the answer. Codon usage bias refers to differences among organisms in the frequency of occurrence of synonymous codons in mRNA. Faster translation rates and higher accuracy is achieved by optimal codons. If the translation rate changes before the process of beta sheet formation is finished, newly synthesized sequence influences the structure earlier (or later) than usual and may have an effect on the folding of the protein as the folding of the beta sheet occurs slower than the alpha helix formation [52]. Translation or protein folding disorders because of ribosome stalling (pause) may occur if the mutation is a change from optimal to less frequent codon. S904S SNP gives rise to less frequent codons, so ribosome stalling can happen. In the case of SNP L679L where the codon with higher codon usage appears, the sheet may not finish creating the structure when the helix appears [53]. As a consequence, kinase activity and/or specificity get changed. These postulated mechanisms are not mutually exclusive [54]. The mutant Y791F reduces the energy of the wild type by 7% and L769L (T > G) variant the by 17%, concluding that the L769L polymorphism reduces the MFE of small *RET* mRNA [45, 55]. Because of its cosegregation of S904S with G691S, the results obtained could be interpreted as a founder effect without influence as genetic modifier [38].

The G691S SNP occurs close to the residue Y687 in the cytoplasmic tail of the RET amidst transmembrane region. Two scenarios are possible to explain the G691S polymorphism exerting an effect in PTC without activation by *RET* rearrangement. *Firstly*, although *RET* expressed in the parafollicular C-cells and hence might influence the microenvironment of the follicular cells [56]. *Alternatively*, the two amino acids, glycine in the wild-type RET protein and serine in the polymorphic *RET* variant, confer different electrochemical and conformational structures to the RET protein, and accordingly effect the subcellular localization, folding, processing or function of the protein [7, 57, 58]. So lot of changes in *RET* proto-oncogene at mRNA level or at protein level can be conferred by single nucleotide polymorphisms that deregulates the *MAP* kinase or Akt pathway, hence predisposing a person to thyroid cancer [18, 45].

6. Patients and controls

Blood samples of 140 cases were collected from thyroid cancer patients attending Department of Nuclear Medicine, at Sher-I-Kashmir Institute of Medical Sciences (SKIMS), besides blood samples were obtained from 180 healthy controls from the Out Patients Departments of SKIMS. The cases and controls gave written pre-informed consent. Questionnaire was used to record demographic and clinico-pathological characteristics of each patient. This study was approved by the Ethical committee of the SKIMS.

0.5 ml of peripheral blood was obtained from each subject in EDTA containing vials (200 µl of 0.5 M, pH = 8.0) and stored at −20°C till use.

7. Genotyping by restriction fragment length polymorphism (PCR-RFLP)

Salting out method was used for the extraction of DNA from blood samples. Automated DNA sequencing of the *RAS* genes revealed one frequent SNP at codon 27 (T81C SNP) of *HRAS*. This SNP along with three other SNPs mentioned above were conducted in our study by PCR-RFLP which is the simple, cheap and common genotyping method.

Restriction enzymes (REs) are called molecular scissors. They recognize and cut specific sequences. The restriction endonuclease type II for SNP detection is selected, such that it recognizes and cleaves one of the polymorphic bases. Upon incubation at optimum temperature and for optimum time with a buffer, the enzyme restricts the DNA, at a specific site. Electrophoresis of the digested products yields fragments of sizes based on the cleavage pattern. If both the alleles harbor the base recognized by the enzyme, fragments of sizes accounting cumulative to the undigested product are obtained (homozygous for that base). If one of the allele harbors a different base, then the single allele is cleaved resulting usually in 3 fragments—the original undigested product, and two digested fragments of sizes cumulatively accounting to the original PCR product (heterozygous). If more than one restriction site is present within the allele, more than two fragments are made from the same allele and the number of fragments depends on number of restriction sites present within the allele. Absence of the base recognized by the enzyme does not result in digestion thereby retaining the original PCR product (Homozygous).

Oligonucleotide Primers and the corresponding Restriction enzymes for codon 691, codon 769, codon 904 of *RET* SNPs along with Annealing temperatures are elucidated **Table 1**. The PCR products were then checked on 2% agarose gel as described earlier.

7.1 Restriction digestion procedure

10 µl of the PCR products were subjected to restriction digestion by *Ban*I, *Taq*I, and *Rsa*I for codons 691,769 and 904 of *RET* SNPs respectively. The reaction conditions were set up according to the supplier of restriction enzymes (**Table 2**). For *RET* codon 691 the homozygous wild type (GG) has one *Ban*I site and is branded by 267 and 187 bp fragments while the (AA) homozygote (variant) offered a single fragment of 454 bp and heterozygous form (G/A) showed 454, 267 and

Amplicon	Primer sequence	A_T (°C)	Product (bp)	RE*	DP** (bp)
HRAS					
Codon 27 (T81C)	F 5′-CAGGAGACCCTGTAGGAGGA-3′ R 5′-GGCACCTGGACGGCGGCGCTAG-3′	60	186	*Dra*III	128 and 58
RET					
Codon 691 (G2071A)	F-5CAGAGCATACGCAGCCTGTAC-3 R-5-GCCTCGTCTGCCCAGCGTTG-3	60	454	*Ban*I	267 and 187
Codon 769 (T2307G)	F-5-CCTGTCCACTGATCCCAAAG-3 R-5-CACTCAGCCCGTGGACTC-3	64	460	*Taq*I	190 and 270
Codon 904 (C2712G)	F-5-GGTCTCACCAGGCCGCTAC-3 R-5-TCGGTATCTTTCCTAGGCTTC-3	62	332	*Rsa*I	224 and 108

RE, restriction enzyme.
***DP, digestion product.*

Table 1.
Conditions and consumables used for screening RET SNPs.

Reagents	Volume (μl)	Incubation
Water	18	Incubation temperature and time for *Ban*I, *Taq*I and *Rsa*I was 37°C for 1–16 h
10× buffer R	2	
PCR product	10	
Restriction enzyme	1	

Table 2.
Composition of RD mixture for codons 691, 769 and 904 of RET.

187 bp. For *RET* codon 769 the homozygous wild type (TT) has one *Taq*I site and is branded by 270 and 190 bp fragments while the (GG) homozygote (variant) offered a single fragment of 460 bp and heterozygous form (T/G) showed 460, 270 and 190 bp. In case of *RET* codon 904 the homozygous wild type (CC) offered a single fragment of 332 bp and the (GG) homozygote (variant) has one *Rsa*I site and is branded by 224 and 108 bp fragments while as heterozygous form (C/G) showed 332, 224 and 108 bp fragments.

The PCR products were visualized on a 3% agarose gel containing 0.5 μg/ml ethidium bromide and photographed.

8. Statistical analysis

Statistical analysis was performed by using SPSS software (V.16.0). Statistical significance was considered when $P \leq 0.05$ [59].

9. Polymorphic analysis of codon G691S, L769L and S904S of *RET* gene

A total of 140 cases (thyroid cancer patients) and 180 normal healthy controls were studied for polymorphic analysis of codon G691S, L769L and S904S of *RET* gene. **Table 3** shows the risk and demographic factors of study group. Mean age and smoking was not having significant differences among cases and controls. The mean age of the controls and patients were 38 ± 14.6 years and 35 ± 13.4 years respectively. Almost 71% (100 of 140) were <45 years of age and 29% (40 of 140) were ≥45 years of age. Only 19% (26 of 140) of the cases were females and 81% (114 of 140) were males. There was a difference between cases and controls with respect to their gender. Only 11% (16 of 140) of thyroid cancer patients were smokers and 89% (124 of 140) were non-smokers with no significant difference between the groups ($P > 0.05$). Based on the histology 84% (118 of 140) of the included cases were papillary thyroid cancers and 16% (22 of 140) were follicular type.

9.1 Analysis of RET codon G691S, L769L and S904S polymorphism

Table 4 represents the genotype distributions of *RET* codon L691S, L769L and S904S polymorphisms in the cases and controls. There was a significant difference in the genotype distributions between cases and controls in all the three polymorphisms ($P < 0.05$) (**Table 4**).

In *RET* G691S (*rs*1799939), the overall dissemination of variant alleles (GA + AA) in cases was 62.9% as compared to 44.5% in controls ($P < 0.05$; OR = 2.1). **Table 5** shows the Link between *RET* G691S phenotypes and clinicopathological characteristics. For further classification, our study found higher distribution of variant alleles (GA + AA) in female cases as equated to healthy controls (63.2 vs. 47%; $P < 0.05$). Higher frequency of variant genotype was found in cases with no smoking status as compare to non-smoker controls (71.4 vs. 42.9%; $P < 0.05$). No significance was found between G691S polymorphism and any other clinicopathological characteristics (**Table 5**).

In *RET* L769L (*rs*1800861), the overall dissemination of variant alleles (TG + GG) in controls 88% as against 70% in cases ($P < 0.05$; OR = 0.3). **Table 6** represents the connection between *RET* L769L phenotypes and clinicopathological characteristics of patients. For further organization, our study found lower distribution of variant alleles (TG + GG) in <45 years old patients as compared to healthy controls (68 vs. 88%; $P < 0.05$). A significant difference was found between variant alleles (TG + GG) of cases (males—61.5%, females—71.9%) and controls (males—89.5%, females—87%) ($P < 0.05$). Non-smoker controls had higher frequency of variant allele as compared to cases with no smoking status (87 vs. 67.7%; $P < 0.05$). A higher frequency of variant alleles (82.1%) (62%) was found in thyroid cancer patients having no history of benign thyroid disease as compared to patients with history of benign thyroid disease (62%; $P < 0.05$). *RET* gene L769L polymorphism was not found to be associated with any other clinicopathological characteristics (**Table 6**).

In *RET* S904S (*rs*1800863), the overall dissemination of variant alleles (CG + GG) in controls was 44% as against 56% in cases ($P < 0.05$; OR = 1.6). **Table 7** lists the connection between *RET* S904S phenotypes and clinicopathological characteristics of study cases and controls. For further arrangement, our study found lower distribution of variant alleles (CG + GG) in controls of ≥45 years of age as compared to matched thyroid cancer cases (28 vs. 45%; $P < 0.05$). We found a higher distribution of variant alleles (CG + GG) in male thyroid cancer patients as compared to healthy controls (69 vs. 57%; $P < 0.05$). A lower frequency of variant alleles was found in thyroid cancer patients having no history of benign thyroid disease when compared to patients having benign thyroid disease (43 vs. 63%; $P < 0.05$). No association was found between any other clinicopathological characteristic and *RET* gene L769L polymorphism (**Table 7**).

Characteristics	**Cases n = 140 (%)**	**Controls n = 180 (%)**	**χ^2-value**	**P value**
Age group				
<45	100 (71)	130 (72)	0.025	>0.05
≥45	40 (29)	50 (28)		
Sex				
Female	114 (81)	104 (58)	20.2	**<0.05**
Male	26 (19)	76 (42)		
Dwelling				
Rural	112 (80)	98 (54.4)	22.8	**<0.05**
Urban	28 (20)	82 (45.6)		
Smoking				
Never	124 (89)	140 (77.8)	6.3	**<0.05**
Ever	16 (11)	40 (22.2)		
Benign thyroid disease				
Yes	84 (60)			
No	56 (40)			
TSH levels				
Elevated	100 (71)			
Normal	40 (29)			
Histological types				
Papillary	118 (84)			
Follicular	22 (16)			
Tumor grade				
WD	134 (96)			
PD	06 (04)			
Stage, <45 years				
Stage I	94(67)			
Stage II	06 (4.3)			
Stage, 45 years				
Stage I and II	36 (25.7)			
Stage III and above	04 (03)			
Vascular/capsular invasion				
Yes	68 (48.5)			
No	72 (51.5)			
Lymph node metastasis				
Yes	52 (37)			
No	88 (63)			

TSH, thyroid stimulating hormone; WD, well differentiated thyroid cancer; PD, poorly differentiated thyroid cancer.

Table 3.
Details of thyroid cancer cases and controls for the study.

SNP	Cases n = 140 (%)	Controls n =180 (%)	OR (95% CI)	P-value
G691S (G2071A)				
Genotype				
GG	52 (37.1)	100 (55.5)	1.0 **(ref.)**	
GA	64 (45.7)	64 (35.5)	1.9 (1.1–3.2)	**<0.05**
AA	24 (17.2)	16 (09)	2.9 (1.2–6.6)	
Allele type				
G	168(60)	264 (73.3)	1.0 **(ref.)**	
A	112(40)	96 (26.7)	1.8 (1.2–2.5)	**<0.05**
L769L (T2307G)				
Genotype				
TT	42 (30)	22 (12)	1.0 **(ref.)**	
TG	70 (50)	110 (61)	0.32 (0.17–0.57)	**<0.05**
GG	28 (20)	48 (27)	0.30 (0.15–0.6)	
Allele type				
T	154(55)	154 (42)	1.0 **(ref.)**	
G	126(45)	206 (58)	0.61 (0.44–0.82)	**<0.05**
S904S (C2712G)				
Genotype				
CC	62 (44)	102 (56)	1.0 **(ref.)**	
CG	64 (46)	70(40)	1.5 (0.93–2.4)	**<0.05**
GG	14 (10)	08 (04)	2.8 (1.1–7.0)	
Allele type				
C	188(67)	274 (76)	1.0 **(ref.)**	
G	92(33)	86 (24)	1.5 (1.0–2.1)	**<0.05**

TSH, thyroid stimulating hormone; WD, well differentiated thyroid cancer; PD, poorly differentiated thyroid cancer; BTD, benign thyroid disease.

Table 4.
Genotype frequencies of cases and controls in RET polymorphisms.

9.2 Mode of inheritance in genetic association studies of RET polymorphisms

The risk of thyroid cancer with respect to gender and smoking status with *RET* G691S (G2071A), L769L (T2307G) and S904S (C2712G) polymorphisms. Recessive, dominant, co-dominant and additive inheritance models were used to assess Adjusted ORs. The inheritance model matching individual SNP data shall have lowest P-value. For *RET* G691S and L769L polymorphism dominant inheritance model is appropriate while as additive inheritance model is appropriate for *RET* S904S polymorphism. The results are presented in **Tables 8–10**.

9.3 Association between RET haplotypes and thyroid cancer risk

In order to evaluate the combined effect of the three polymorphisms on thyroid cancer risk Haplotype analyses were conducted. Among both cases and controls all haplotypes have frequencies >5%. G2071/2307G/ C2712 (GGC) was the most

	Cases n (%)	GG n (%)	GA + AA n (%)	Controls n (%)	GG n (%)	GA + AA n (%)	OR (95% CI)	P value
Overall genotype	n = 140	52 (37.1)	88 (62.9)	n = 180	100 (55.5)	80 (44.5)	2.1 (1.3–3.2)	<0.05
Age group								
<45	100 (71)	30 (30)	70 (70)	130 (72)	62 (48)	68 (52)	2.1 (1.2–3.6)	**<0.05**
≥45	40 (29)	22 (55)	18 (45)	50 (28)	38 (76)	12 (24)	2.6 (3.6–6.2)	**<0.05**
Sex								
Female	114 (81)	42 (36.8)	72 (63.2)	104 (58)	60 (58)	44 (42)	2.3 (1.3–3.9)	**<0.05**
Male	26 (19)	10 (38.5)	16 (61.5)	76 (42)	40 (53)	36 (47)	1.8 (0.72–4.4)	>0.05
Dwelling								
Rural	112 (80)	44 (39.3)	68 (60.7)	98 (54.4)	56 (57.1)	42 (42.9)	2.0 (1.2–3.4)	**<0.05**
Urban	28 (20)	08 (28.5)	20 (71.5)	82 (45.6)	44 (53.6)	38 (46.4)	2.9 (1.1–7.2)	**<0.05**
Smoking								
Never	124 (89)	42 (28.6)	82 (71.4)	140 (77.8)	80 (57.1)	60 (42.9)	2.6 (1.5–4.5)	**<0.05**
Ever	16 (11)	10 (62.5)	06 (37.5)	40 (22.2)	20 (50)	20 (50)	0.6 (0.1–2.8)	>0.05
BTD								
Yes	84 (60)	30 (35.7)	54 (64.2)					
No	56 (40)	22 (39.2)	34 (60.8)				1.2 (0.8–1.9)	>0.05
TSH levels								
Elevated	100 (71)	40 (40)	60 (60)					
Normal	40 (29)	12 (30)	28 (70)				0.6 (0.2–1.5)	>0.05
Histological types								
Papillary	118(84)	44(37.2)	74(62.8)					
Follicular	22(16)	08(36.3)	14(63.7)				1.0 (0.3–3.2)	>0.05
Tumor grade								
WD	134 (96)	50 (37.3)	84 (62.7)					
PD	06 (04)	02 (33.3)	04 (66.7)				0.8 (0.06–9.7)	>0.05
Stage, <45 years								
Stage I	94 (67)	28 (29.7)	66 (70.3)					
Stage II	06 (4.3)	02 (33.3)	04 (66.7)				1.2 (0.1–15.3)	>0.05
Stage, 45 years								
Stage I and II	36 (25.7)	20 (55.5)	16 (44.5)					
Stage III and above	04 (03)	02 (50)	02 (50)				0.8 (0.09–6.3)	>0.05
Vascular/ capsular invasion								
Yes	68 (48.5)	22 (32.3)	46 (67.7)					
No	72 (51.5)	30 (41.6)	42 (58.4)				1.5 (0.75–3)	>0.05
Lymph node metastasis								

	Cases n (%)	GG n (%)	GA + AA n (%)	Controls n (%)	GG n (%)	GA + AA n (%)	OR (95% CI)	P value
Yes	52 (37)	18 (34.6)	34 (65.4)					
No	88 (63)	34 (38.6)	54 (61.4)				1.2 (0.5–2.7)	>0.05

TSH, thyroid stimulating hormone; WD, well differentiated thyroid cancer; PD, poorly differentiated thyroid cancer; BTD, benign thyroid disease.

Table 5.
Clinicopathological characteristics vs. RET G691S (G2071A) genotypes.

	Cases n (%)	TT n (%)	TG + GG n (%)	Controls n (%)	TT n (%)	TG + GG n (%)	OR (95% CI)	P value
Overall genotype	n = 140	42 (30)	98 (70)	n = 180	22 (12)	158 (88)	0.3 (0.17–0.6)	**<0.05**
Age group								
<45	100 (71)	32 (32)	68 (68)	130 (72)	16 (12)	114 (88)	0.3 (0.14–0.5)	**<0.05**
≥45	40 (29)	10 (25)	30 (75)	50 (28)	06 (12)	44 (88)	0.4 (0.13–1.2)	>0.05
Sex								
Female	114 (81)	32 (28.0)	82 (71.9)	104 (58)	14 (13)	90 (87)	0.4 (0.18–0.85)	**<0.05**
Male	26 (19)	10 (38.4)	16 (61.5)	76 (42)	08 (10.5)	68 (89.5)	0.2 (0.07–0.6)	**<0.05**
Dwelling								
Rural	112 (80)	36 (32.1)	76 (67.8)	98 (54)	10 (10)	88 (90)	0.23 (0.1–0.5)	**<0.05**
Urban	28 (20)	06 (21.4)	22 (78.5)	82 (46)	12 (15)	70(85)	0.6 (0.2–1.8)	>0.05
Smoking								
Never	124 (89)	40 (32.2)	84 (67.7)	140 (78)	18 (13)	122 (87)	0.3 (0.16–0.55)	**<0.05**
Ever	16 (11)	02 (12.5)	14 (87.5)	40 (22)	04 (10)	36 (90)	1.1 (0.16–6.2)	>0.05
BTD								
Yes	84 (60)	32 (38)	52 (62)				0.35(0.15–0.78)	**<0.05**
No	56 (40)	10 (17.8)	46 (82.1)					
TSH levels								
Elevated	100 (71)	30 (30)	70 (70)				0.25(0.1–0.62)	>0.05
Normal	40 (29)	12 (30)	28 (70)					
Histological types								
Papillary	118 (84)	36 (30.5)	82 (69.4)				0.85 (0.3–2.2)	>0.05
Follicular	22 (16)	06 (27.2)	16 (72.7)					
Tumor grade								
WD	134 (96)	40 (29.8)	94 (70.14)				1.17 (0.19–6.5)	>0.05
PD	06 (04)	02 (33.3)	04 (66.6)					
Stage, <45 years								
Stage I	94 (67)	28 (29.8)	66 (70.2)				4.7 (0.8–26.8)	>0.05

	Cases n (%)	TT n (%)	TG + GG n (%)	Controls n (%)	TT n (%)	TG + GG n (%)	OR (95% CI)	P value
Stage II	06 (4.3)	04 (66.6)	02 (33.3)					
Stage, 45 years								
Stage I and II	36 (25.7)	08 (22.2)	28 (77.8)				3.5 (0.42–28.7)	>0.05
Stage III and above	04 (03)	02 (50)	02 (50)					
Vascular/ capsular invasion								
Yes	68 (48.5)	22 (32.3)	46 (67.7)				0.8 (0.4–1.6)	>0.05
No	72 (51.5)	20 (27.8)	52 (72.2)					
Lymph node metastasis								
Yes	52 (37)	18 (34.6)	34 (65.4)				0.7 (0.32–1.4)	>0.05
No	88 (63)	24 (27.2)	64 (72.8)					

TSH, thyroid stimulating hormone; WD, well differentiated thyroid cancer; PD, poorly differentiated thyroid cancer; BTD, benign thyroid disease.

Table 6.
Clinicopathological characteristics vs. RET L769L (T2307G) genotypes.

	Cases n (%)	CC n (%)	CG + GG n (%)	Controls n (%)	CC n (%)	CG + GG n (%)	OR (95% CI)	P-value
Overall genotype	n = 140	62 (44)	78 (56)	n = 180	102 (56)	78 (44)	1.6 (1.0–2.4)	**<0.05**
Age group								
<45	100 (71)	40 (64.5)	60 (35.5)	130 (72)	66 (51)	64 (49)	1.5 (0.9–2.9)	>0.05
≥45	40 (29)	22 (55)	18 (45)	50 (28)	36 (72)	14 (28)	2.1 (0.84–5.0)	**<0.05**
Sex								
Female	114 (81)	54 (47)	60 (53)	104 (58)	58 (56)	46 (44)	1.4 (0.8–2.4)	>0.05
Male	26 (19)	08 (31)	18 (69)	76 (42)	44 (43)	32 (57)	3.1 (1.2–8.0)	**<0.05**
Dwelling								
Rural	112 (80)	46 (41)	66(59)	98 (54)	54 (55)	44 (45)	1.7 (0.96–2.9)	>0.05
Urban	28 (20)	16 (57)	12(43)	82 (46)	48 (58.5)	34 (41.5)	1.05 (0.4–2.4)	>0.05
Smoking								
Never	124 (89)	56 (45)	68 (55)	140 (78)	78 (56)	62 (44)	1.5 (0.9–2.4)	>0.05
Ever	16 (11)	06 (37.5)	10 (62.5)	40 (22)	24 (60)	16 (40)	2.5 (0.75–8.2)	>0.05
BTD								
Yes	84 (60)	30 (36)	54 (64)					
No	56 (40)	32 (57)	24 (43)				2.4 (1.2–4.8)	**<0.05**
TSH levels								
Elevated	100 (71)	40 (40)	60 (60)					
Normal	40 (29)	22 (55)	18 (45)				1.8 (0.7–3.7)	>0.05
Histological types								
Papillary	118 (84)	56 (47)	62 (53)					

	Cases n (%)	CC n (%)	CG + GG n (%)	Controls n (%)	CC n (%)	CG + GG n (%)	OR (95% CI)	P-value
Follicular	22 (16)	06 (27)	16 (73)				0.4 (0.15–1.08)	>0.05
Tumor grade								
WD	134 (96)	60 (45)	74 (55)					
PD	06 (04)	02 (33)	04 (67)				0.6 (0.10–3.4)	>0.05
Stage, < 45 years								
Stage I	94 (67)	40 (42.5)	54 (57.5)					
Stage II	06 (4.3)	02 (33)	04 (67)				0.7 (0.12–4.0)	>0.05
Stage, 45 years								
Stage I and II	36 (25.7)	18 (50)	18 (50)					
Stage III and above	04 (03)	02 (50)	02 (50)				1.0 (0.12–7.9)	>0.05
Vascular/ capsular invasion								
Yes	68 (48.5)	32 (47)	36 (53)					
No	72 (51.5)	30 (41.7)	42 (58.3)				0.8 (0.4–1.56)	>0.05
Lymph node metastasis								
Yes	52 (37)	28 (54)	24 (46)					
No	88 (63)	34 (39)	54 (61)				0.5 (0.25–1.0)	>0.05

TSH, thyroid stimulating hormone; WD, well differentiated thyroid cancer; PD, poorly differentiated thyroid cancer; BTD, benign thyroid disease.

Table 7.
Clinicopathological characteristics vs. RET S904S (C2712G) genotypes.

Genotypes and alleles (patients vs. controls)	Cases (n = 140)	Controls (n = 180)	OR (95% CI)	P value
Recessive model (AA vs. GA + GG)				
GA + GG	116	164	1.0 **(ref.)**	
AA	24	16	2.12 (1.0–4.7)	0.027
Dominant model (AA+ GA vs. GG)				
GG	52	100	1.0 **(ref.)**	
AA + GA	88	80	2.11 (1.3–3.3)	**0.001**
Co-dominant model (GA vs. AA + GG)				
AA + GG	76	116	1.0 **(ref.)**	
GA	64	64	1.5 (1.0–2.3)	0.066
Additive model (AA vs. GG)				
GG	52	100	1.0 **(ref.)**	
AA	24	16	2.8 (1.4–5.7)	0.003

Table 8.
G691S (G2071A) polymorphism association with thyroid cancer.

Genotypes and alleles (patients vs. controls)	Cases (n = 140)	Controls (n = 180)	OR (95% CI)	P value
Recessive model (GG vs. TG + TT)				
TG + TT	112	132	1.0 **(ref.)**	
GG	28	48	0.7 (0.4–1.2)	0.17
Dominant model (GG + TG vs. TT)				
TT	42	22	1.0 **(ref.)**	
GG + TG	98	158	0.32 (0.2–0.6)	**0.000**
Co-dominant model (TG vs. GG + TT)				
GG + TT	70	70	1.0 **(ref.)**	
TG	70	110	0.63 (0.4–1.0)	0.047
Additive model (GG vs. TT)				
TT	42	22	1.0 **(ref.)**	
GG	28	48	0.3 (0.15–0.6)	0.001

Table 9.
Genetic model for L769L (T2307G) polymorphism.

common haplotype, with frequencies of 24% in cases and 33% in controls. The complete dissemination of various haplotypes between cases and controls presented a clear difference (P < 0.0001). Haplotype pattern for the three SNPs is shown in **Table 11**. Haplotypes with frequency <1% was omitted from the study. After stratified by gender, age and smoking status the haplotype frequencies were estimated from the genotyping data. In our study, the most common haplotype is taken

Genotypes and alleles (patients vs. controls)	Cases (n = 140)	Controls (n = 180)	OR (95% CI)	P-value
Recessive model (GG vs. CG + CC)				
CG + CC	126	172	1.0 **(ref.)**	
GG	14	08	2.4 **(0.97–5.8)**	0.051
Dominant model (GG + CG vs. CC)				
CC	62	102	1.0 **(ref.)**	
GG + CG	78	78	1.64 (1.0–2.6)	0.028
Co-dominant model (CG vs. GG + CC)				
GG + CC	76	110	1.0 **(ref.)**	
CG	64	70	1.3 (0.8–2.0)	0.22
Additive model (GG vs. CC)				
CC	62	102	1.0 **(ref.)**	
GG	14	08	2.8 (1.1–7.2)	**0.021**

Table 10.
Genetic model for S904S (C2712G) polymorphism.

G2071A	T2307G	C2712G	Total frequency	Cases	Controls	Cumulative frequency	OR (95% CI)	P value
G	G	C	0.3061	0.2498	0.3337	0.3061	1.00 (ref)	–
G	T	C	0.2122	0.2004	0.2321	0.5183	0.94 (0.48–1.84)	0.86
A	G	C	0.1224	0.1084	0.1503	0.6407	1.26 (0.55–2.87)	0.59
A	T	G	0.0999	0.1442	0.0657	0.7406	**0.24 (0.10–0.57)**	**0.0012**
A	T	C	0.0843	0.1129	0.0506	0.8249	**0.38 (0.17–0.83)**	**0.016**
G	T	G	0.0817	0.0925	0.0738	0.9066	**0.23 (0.08–0.64)**	**0.0051**
G	G	G	0.075	0.0573	0.0938	0.9816	1.59 (0.59–4.31)	0.36
A	G	G	0.0184	0.0345	0	1	0.05 (0.00–1.37)	0.076

The OR (95% CI) of thyroid cancer associated with each haplotype was estimated by comparison with the common reference haplotype. ref: reference.

Table 11.
Haplotype frequencies and its association with thyroid cancer.

as the reference group and haplotype-specific ORs are estimated by the haplotype-based logistic regression method [60]. The frequencies for the estimated 3-marker haplotypes among patients and controls are shown in **Table 11.**

10. Conclusion

Thyroid tumors signify a proper model for the study of epithelial neoplastic transformation. At the genomic level, thyroid cancers gather a number of changes and it has been projected that genomic instability has a vital role in the development of thyroid neoplasms [61].

With erudite genetic tools producing a treasure of information, we have added improved vision into the mechanisms driving thyroid tumor development. Recognition of these features is crucial to the management of patients with TC. New therapeutics is being designed based on our improved understanding of this disease course.

In Kashmiri population we studied genetic alterations of *RET* genes in thyroid cancer patients. Following are the major findings of our study;

- In *RET* G691S (*rs*1799939), the total distribution of variant alleles (CA + AA) in controls was 44.5% as against 62.9% in controls which revealed a 2-fold higher risk of variant allele (TC + CC) in cases against the controls ($P < 0.05$).

- In *RET* L769L (*rs*1800861), the total distribution of variant alleles (TG + GG) in controls was 88% as against 70% in cases ($P < 0.05$; OR = 0.3).

- In *RET* S904S (*rs*1800863), the total distribution of variant alleles (CG + GG) in controls was 44% as against 56% in cases ($P < 0.05$; OR = 1.6).

- We found higher distribution of variant alleles (CG + GG) in TC cases of ≥45 years of age and male gender (45 and 69%) as compared to matched healthy controls (28 and 57%) ($P < 0.05$). Association was also observed with BTD ($P < 0.05$).

- *RET* G691S and L769L polymorphisms follow "*Dominant inheritance model*" while as "*Additive inheritance model*" is appropriate for analysis of *RET* S904S polymorphism.

- In *RET* codon G691S, L769L and S904S polymorphism the most over-represented haplotype is A T G followed by G T G and A T C depending upon their Akaike information criteria (P-value).

In conclusion, our study shows that among different polymorphisms predisposing to thyroid tumors, *RET* gene polymorphism is among the prominent ones. Our results support the earlier reports of the G691S/S904S polymorphism in *RET* gene as a marked predisposing factor for the risk of developing thyroid tumors in our population with G691S variant showing an increased risk for the non-smokers but this needs to be authenticated in a large sample study in the future to determine the course of thyroid cancer. Further we conclude L769L polymorphism to be protective in our series of thyroid cancer patients. Apart from it our data suggest that some specific haplotypes (A T G, G T G, and A T C) of *RET* are over-represented and may act as low penetrance alleles in the predisposition to thyroid cancer.

Author details

Syed Mudassar[1*†], Mosin S. Khan[1†], Shariq R. Masoodi[2], Mahboob Ul Hussain[3] and Khurshid I. Andrabi[3]

1 Department of Clinical Biochemistry, Sher-I-Kashmir Institute of Medical Sciences, Srinagar, Kashmir, India

2 Department of Endocrinology, Sher-I-Kashmir Institute of Medical Sciences, Srinagar, Kashmir, India

3 Department of Biotechnology, University of Kashmir, Srinagar, Kashmir, India

*Address all correspondence to: syed.mudassar@skims.ac.in

†Both authors (first two) have contributed equally.

IntechOpen

© 2019 The Author(s). Licensee IntechOpen. This chapter is distributed under the terms of the Creative Commons Attribution License (http://creativecommons.org/licenses/by/3.0), which permits unrestricted use, distribution, and reproduction in any medium, provided the original work is properly cited.

References

[1] Corner J, Bailey C. Cancer Nursing Care in Context. Oxford: Blackwell Publishing; 2001

[2] Yarbro C, Frogge M, Goodman M. Cancer Nursing: Principles and Practice. 6th ed. Boston, MA: Jones and Bartlett Publishers; 2005

[3] Sarlis NJ, Benvenga S. Molecular signaling in thyroid cancer. Cancer Treatment and Research. 2004;**122**: 237-264

[4] Sarlis NJ. Expression patterns of cellular growth-controlling genes in non-medullary thyroid cancer: Basic aspects. Reviews in Endocrine and Metabolic Disorders. 2000;**1**:183-196

[5] Hundahl SA, Fleming ID, Fremgen AM, Menck HR. A National Cancer Data Base report on 53,856 cases of thyroid carcinoma treated in the U.S., 1985–1995. Cancer. 1998;**83**:2638-2648

[6] Grogan RH, Mitmaker EJ, Clark OH. The evolution of biomarkers in thyroid cancer-from mass screening to a personalized biosignature. Cancers. 2010;**2**:885-912

[7] Bunone G, Uggeri M, Mondellini P, et al. RET receptor expression in thyroid follicular epithelial cell-derived tumors. Cancer Research. 2000;**60**:2845-2849

[8] Santoro M et al. Ret oncogene activation in human thyroid neoplasms is restricted to the papillary cancer subtype. The Journal of Clinical Investigation. 1992;**89**:1517-1522

[9] Grieco M, Santoro M, et al. PTC is a novel rearranged form of the ret protooncogene and is frequently detected in vivo in human thyroid papillary carcinomas. Cell. 1990;**60**:557-563

[10] Santoro M et al. Molecular characterization of RET/PTC3: A novel rearranged version of the RET proto-oncogene in a human thyroid papillary carcinoma. Oncogene. 1994;**9**:509-516

[11] Eng C. RET proto-oncogene in the development of human cancer. Journal of Clinical Oncology. 1999;**17**:380-393

[12] Tallini G, Asa SL. RET oncogene activation in papillary thyroid carcinoma. Advances in Anatomic Pathology. 2001;**8**:345-354

[13] Fenton CL, Lukes Y, Nicholson D, et al. The RET/PTC mutations are common in sporadic papillary thyroid carcinoma of children and young adults. The Journal of Clinical Endocrinology and Metabolism. 2000;**85**:1170-1175

[14] Nikiforov YE. Molecular analysis of thyroid tumors. Modern Pathology. 2011;**24**:S34-S43

[15] Frazer KA et al. A second generation human haplotype map of over 3.1 million SNPs. Nature. 2007;**449**:851-861

[16] Stephens LA, Powell NG, Grubb SJ, Jeremiah JA, et al. Investigation of loss of heterozygosity and SNP frequencies in the RET gene in papillary thyroid carcinoma. Thyroid. 2005;**15**:100-105

[17] Adjadj E, Schlumberger M, de Vathaire F. Germ-line DNA polymorphisms and susceptibility to differentiated thyroid cancer. The Lancet Oncology. 2009;**10**:181-190

[18] Fitze G, Schreiber M, Kuhlisch E, Schackert HK, et al. Association of RET protooncogene codon 45 polymorphism with Hirschsprung disease. American Journal of Human Genetics. 1999;**65**: 1469-1473

[19] Borrego S, Ruiz A, Saez ME, Gimm O, Gao X, Lopez-Alonso M, et al. RET genotypes comprising specific

haplotypes of polymorphic variants predispose to isolated Hirschsprung disease. Journal of Medical Genetics. 2000;**37**:572-578

[20] Lesueur F, Corbex M, McKay JD, et al. Specific haplotypes of the RET proto-oncogene are over-represented in patients with sporadic papillary thyroid carcinoma. Journal of Medical Genetics. 2002;**39**:260-265

[21] Ho T, Li G, Zhao C, Wei Q, Sturgis EM. RET polymorphisms and haplotypes and risk of differentiated thyroid cancer. Laryngoscope. 2005;**115**: 1035-1041

[22] Pandith AA, Siddiqi MA. Burden of cancers in the valley of Kashmir: 5 year epidemiological study reveals a different scenario. Tumor Biology. 2012;**33**: 1629-1637

[23] Kleiman DA, Buitrago D, Crowley MJ, Housman D. Human DNA polymorphism. The New England Journal of Medicine. 1995;**332**:318-320

[24] The International Hap Map Consortium. The International Hap Map project. Nature. 2003;**426**:789-796

[25] Takahashi M, Ritz J, Cooper GM. Activation of a novel human transforming gene, ret, by DNA rearrangement. Cell. 1985;**42**:581-588

[26] Takahashi M, Buma Y, et al. Cloning and expression of the ret proto-oncogene encoding a tyrosine kinase with two potential transmembrane domains. Oncogene. 1988;**3**:571-578

[27] Pachnis V, Mankoo B, Costantini F. Expression of the c-ret proto-oncogene during mouse embryogenesis. Development. 1993;**119**:1005-1017

[28] Tsuzuki T, Takahashi M, Asai N, Iwashita T, Matsuyama M, Asai J. Spatial and temporal expression of the retproto-oncogene product in embryonic, infant and adult rat tissues. Oncogene. 1995;**10**:191-198

[29] Tahira T, Ishizaka Y, Itoh F, Sugimura T, Nagao M. Characterization of ret proto-oncogene mRNAs encoding two isoforms of the protein product in a human neuroblastoma cell line. Oncogene. 1990;**5**:97-102

[30] Myers SM, Eng C, Ponder BA, Mulligan LM. Characterization of RET proto-oncogene splicing variants and polyadenylation sites: A novel C-terminus for RET. Oncogene. 1995;**11**: 2039-2045

[31] Jing S, Wen D, Yu Y, Holst PL, Luo Y, Fang M, et al. GDNF-induced activation of the ret protein tyrosine kinase is mediated by GDNFR-alpha, a novel receptor for GDNF. Cell. 1996;**85**: 1113-1124

[32] Treanor JJ, Goodman L, et al. Characterization of a multicomponent receptor for GDNF. Nature. 1996;**382**: 80-83

[33] Baloh RH, Tansey MG, Lampe PA, Fahrner TJ, et al. Artemin, a novel member of the GDNF ligand family, supports peripheral and central neurons and signals through the GFR alpha3–RET receptor complex. Neuron. 1998;**21**: 1291-1302

[34] Milbrandt J, de Sauvage FJ, Fahrner TJ, et al. Persephin, a novel neurotrophic factor related to GDNF and neurturin. Neuron. 1998;**20**:245-253

[35] Baumgartner-Parzer SM, Lang R, Wagner L, et al. Polymorphisms in exon 13 and intron 14 of the RET protooncogene: Genetic modifiers of medullary thyroid carcinoma? Journal of Clinical Endocrinology and Metabolism. 2005;**90**:6232-6236

[36] Cebrian A, Lesueur F, Martin S, et al. Polymorphisms in the initiators of RET (rearranged during transfection)

signaling pathway and susceptibility to sporadic medullary thyroid carcinoma. Journal of Clinical Endocrinology and Metabolism. 2005; **90**:6268-6274

[37] Machens A, Frank-Raue K, Lorenz K, Rondot S, Raue F, Dralle H. Clinical relevance of RET variants G691S, L769L, S836S and S904S to sporadic medullary thyroid cancer. Clinical Endocrinology. 2012;**76**:691-697

[38] Robledo M et al. Polymorphisms G691S/S904S of RET as genetic modifiers of MEN 2A. Cancer Research. 2003;**63**:1814-1817

[39] Elisei R, Cosci B, Romei C, Bottici V, Sculli M, Lari R, et al. RET exon 11 (G691S) polymorphism is significantly more frequent in sporadic medullary thyroid carcinoma than in the general population. The Journal of Clinical Endocrinology and Metabolism. 2004; **89**:3579-3584

[40] McWhinney SR et al. Intronic single nucleotide polymorphisms in the RET protoonco gene are associated with a subset of apparently sporadic pheochromocytoma and may modulate age of onset. The Journal of Clinical Endocrinology and Metabolism. 2003; **88**(10):4911-4916

[41] Fitze G et al. Functional haplotypes of the RET proto-oncogene promoter are associated with Hirschsprung disease (HSCR). Human Molecular Genetics. 2003;**12**:3207-3214

[42] Garcia-Barcelo M et al. TTF-1 and RET promoter SNPs: Regulation of RET transcription in Hirschsprung's disease. Human Molecular Genetics. 2005;**14**: 191-204

[43] Burzynski GM et al. Identifying candidate Hirschsprung disease associated RET variants. American Journal of Human Genetics. 2005;**76**: 850-858

[44] Plaza-Menacho I, Burzynski GM, de Groot JW, et al. Activated ras and ret oncogenes induce over-expression of cmet (hepatocyte growth factor receptor) in human thyroid epithelialcells. Oncogene. 1997;**14**: 2417-2423

[45] Borrego S, Saez ME, Ruiz A, Gimm O, Lopez-Alonso M, Antiñolo G, et al. Specific polymorphisms in the RET proto-oncogene are over-represented in patients with Hirschsprung disease and may represent loci modifying phenotypic expression. Journal of Medical Genetics. 1999;**36**:771-774

[46] Gil L, Azanedo M, et al. Genetic analysis of RET, GFR alpha 1 and GDNF genes in Spanish families with multiple endocrine neoplasia type 2A. International Journal of Cancer. 2002; **99**:299-304

[47] Tsui-Pierchala BA, Milbrandt J, Johnson EM. NGF utilizes c-Ret via a novel GFL-independent, inter-RTK signaling mechanism to maintain the trophic status of mature sympathetic neurons. Neuron. 2002;**33**:261-273

[48] Sipple JH. The association of pheochromocytoma with carcinoma of the thyroid gland. The American Journal of Medicine. 1961;**31**:163-166

[49] Borrego S, Eng C, Sánchez B, Sáez ME, Navarro E, Antiñolo G. Molecular analysis of RET and GDNF genes in a family with multiple endocrine neoplasia type 2A and Hirschsprung disease. The Journal of Clinical Endocrinology and Metabolism. 1998; **83**:3361-3364

[50] Parmley JL, Hurt LD. How do synonymous mutations affect fitness? Bioassay. 2007;**29**:515-519

[51] Kimchi-Sarfaty C, Oh JM, Kim IW, Sauna ZE, Calcagno AM, Ambudkar SV, et al. A "silent" polymorphisms in the

MDR1 gene changes substrate specificity. Science. 2007;**26**:525-528

[52] Muñoz V, Thompson PA, Hofrichter J, Eaton WA. Folding dynamics and mechanism of β-hairpin formation. Nature. 1997;**390**:196-199

[53] Nakamura Y, Gojobori T, Ikemura T. Codon usage tabulated fromthe international DNA sequence databases. Nucleic Acids Research. 2007;**26**: 334-340

[54] Sromek M, Czetwertyńska M, et al. The frequency of selected polymorphic variants of the RET gene in patients with medullary thyroid carcinoma and in the general population of Central Poland. Endocrine Pathology. 2010;**21**: 178-185

[55] Ceolin L, Siqueira DR, et al. Additive effect of RET polymorphisms on sporadic medullary thyroid carcinoma susceptibility and tumor aggressiveness. European Journal of Endocrinology. 2012;**11**:1-29

[56] Fabien N, Paulin C, Santoro M, Berger N, et al. Detection of RET oncogene activation in human papillary thyroid carcinomas by in situ hybridisation. British Journal of Cancer. 1992;**66**:1094-1098

[57] Fluge O, Haugen DR, Akslen LA, Marstad A, et al. Expression and alternative splicing of c-ret RNA in papillary thyroid carcinomas. Oncogene. 2001;**20**:885-892

[58] Leviev I, Negro F, James RW. Two alleles of the human paraoxonase gene produce different amounts of mRNA. An explanation for differences in serum concentrations of paraoxonase associated with the (Leu-Met54) polymorphism. Arteriosclerosis, Thrombosis, and Vascular Biology. 1997;**17**:2935-2939

[59] Rao J, Scott A. On chi-squared tests for multiway contingency tables with cell proportions estimated from survey data. The Annals of Statistics. 1984;**12**: 46-60

[60] Akaike H. Information measures and model selection. Bulletin of the International Statistical Institute. 1983; **50**:277-290

[61] Sobrinho-Simoes M et al. Molecular pathology of well-differentiated thyroid carcinomas. Virchows Archiv. 2005; **447**:787-793